Mercy, Mandates, Merger

Beth Israel Deaconess Medical Center

Barbara Schwartz

Cambridge Books

Mercy, Mandates, Merger: Beth Israel Deaconess Medical Center
Barbara Schwartz

1. Title   2. Author   3. Medicine/History

Library of Congress Control Number: 2009902938

ISBN : 978-0-615-28720-1

For Lou who gave me a life.
Michael, Larry and William made it worth living.
Elizabeth and Jacob taught me to read.

Barbara Stewart

Table of Contents

Acknowledgments

This book is a memoir of two medical institutions whose mandates were to create the best possible medical care for all, regardless of race or creed.

It was my good fortune to have met each person who helped me with this book. Not only did they share their knowledge, stories, memories and enthusiasm for this project but they demonstrated that we are all members of the Beth Israel Deaconess family.

Were it not for the support of my own family—Michael, Larry, William, Carol and Denise—this book would have remained a wish.

I'm grateful for the interest and encouragement of Dr. Mitchell Rabkin, Mr. Paul Levy, Joyce Clifford, Rabbi Terry Bard, Ruth Freiman and Dr. William Silen—my first interviewees to welcome me into the family. Anthony Lloyd, David Dolins, Sandra Fenwick and

Jack Kasden had the vision and intellect to fulfill the dream. Beryl Chapman and Beverly Singer, early graduates of the Beth Israel School of Nursing, regaled me with humorous stories and pictures in their Plebe uniforms.

Dr. Albert and Nancy Cohen, dear friends, asked weekly, "So, how's the book doing?"

Dr. Paul Dinsmore, psychiatrist, has been a colleague and friend for more than thirty years. His instant availability and sound counsel was of incalcuable value.

Dr. Beth Lown, poet, educator, physician and dear friend, and Dr. Charles Hatem, chaired professor at Harvard, consider medical student training their *raison de'tre*. Drs. Kim Saal, Roger Lange, Clint Koufman and Beth Goldman are my family's team and are always responsive to a call and generous with their time. Dr. Roman Desanctis, cardiologist to kings, has been a friend for decades and prolonged Lou's life.

Dean Daniel Tosteson not only spoke openly and truthfully about the trials and tribulations confronting the Harvard hospitals; his commitment to the survival of Beth Israel was crystal clear.

My sincere gratitude to all my friends and colleagues who not only provided encouragement but day-to-day support. Patricia Ruopp, my cousin and friend, made certain we dined at every new four-star restaurant in Boston and had the best seats in the theaters. Linda Hartling and Kathy Butler Jones, dear friends and published authors, were my cheerleaders. Marcel and Lizanne Cormier kept my old house dry and well lit and drew the etchings of the Beth Israel and Deaconess buildings circa 1928.

Mary Barton, a technologically sophisticated editor, not only embraced the project but made it into a real book. Dr. Leo and Jeanne Stolbach kept me supplied with homegrown tomatoes.

Rosalina Heredia consoled me when my computer skills failed and Leo Henniger was on instant call for computer glitches.

Barbara Beckwith, mentor and editor, generously took the time to teach me punctuation and the difference between muck-raking and journalism. Jim Grace, attorney for the arts, walked me through the permission and copyright process. Violet Linnenthal was so kind to grant me permission to use her husband's book, *First a Dream*, as my Bible. Dr. Bennett Gurian, a geriatric psychia-trist, understood as early as the 1970s the unique problems and medical issues confronting the elderly.

Forty-five people were interviewed and each enriched the story of the Beth Israel Deaconess. Laura Avakian, Jeanette Clough, Lynn Kargman and Francis Friedman, the first woman on the Beth Israel board, all made meaningful contributions.

Mr. Marvin Schorr, president emeritus of the Deaconess board, engaged in an open, honest discussion of the complications of the merger. Mr. Don Lowery shared and clarified, without reserve, many issues that led to the merger. Helaine Miller was a fundraiser *par excellence*. Karen Posnick, Joyce Clifford's senior administrator for decades, provided a history of the nursing department.

Mr. Irving Rabb was chairman of the board in the earlier years of the Beth Israel. As a young man, after his full-time day job, he volunteered his time at night to prep male patients for surgery. Attorney Allan Rottenberg, prior president of the board, described himself as impartial, saying that he is "a compromiser and can see all sides of an issue."

Paul Levy, president and CEO of BIDMC, is not only innovative but decisive, resolute and unable to be intimidated. He said he doesn't second guess himself: If plan A doesn't work, B, C and D are accessible. Successful in cleaning up Boston Harbor, he was well equipped to rescue BIDMC. When interviewed, he said he makes "few promises and fulfills them: I can do anything I put my mind to."

My sincere appreciation goes to each and every one.

Doctors

They work with herbs
and penicillin.
They work with gentleness
and the scalpel.
They dig out the cancer,
close the incision
and say a prayer
to the poverty of the skin.
They are not Gods
though they would like to be;
they are only human
trying to fix up a human.
Many humans die.
They die like the tender,
palpitating berries
in November.
But all along the doctors remember:
First do no harm.
They would kiss if it would heal.
It would not heal.

If the doctors cure
then the sun sees it.
If the doctors kill
than the earth hides it.
The doctors should fear arrogance
more than cardiac arrest.
If they are too proud,
and some are,
then they leave home on horseback
but God returns them on foot.

—Anne Sexton

Chapter One

The Cost of Staying Alive

"The great thing in this world is not so much where we stand
as in what direction we are moving."
—Oliver Wendell Holmes

Once upon a time, health care in America conformed to the Norman Rockwell image of medicine. Community hospitals and dedicated professionals tended to the sick and the poor regardless of their financial resources or social status. Today the ever-escalating cost of health care clouds this nostalgic memory. The focus of the healthcare system has shifted from individual medical needs to money.

Most of us grew up taking health care access for granted. We thought of it as one of our inalienable rights. Many remember when the local family doctor was responsible for all our medical needs and knew us well, having been our family's sole provider of medical care. A few who read this today may be old enough to recall the generation of physicians who made house calls and provided personalized family care in our own homes.

When Dr. Israel Kaufman, our family doctor, came through our front door in Brooklyn, he brought a palpable aura: An important man had arrived. Even before taking off his overcoat, he would ask, "So what happened?" or "What's new?" With all family members from babies to grandparents under his care, there were no secrets. He'd sit down on the green velvet couch for a cup of tea with whoever was in the house—not only to observe a social amenity but as part of the sort of holistic health assessment an old-school physician had time to provide and patients had come to expect.

Dr. Kaufman's armamentarium was limited: It all fit into his small, scuffed, black bag. But his warmth, wisdom and presence made you feel certain that you would recover from whatever ailed you. His prescriptions were few and simple—calamine lotion for a rash, chicken soup with *challah* (a braided bread), castor oil for stomach problems and aspirin to treat a multitude of symptoms. His compensation of two dollars a visit concerned him far less than his mission to care and to heal.

Perhaps this is an idealization. Yet, I think not. He was our respected family doctor who provided an essential service and abided by the caveat of the Hippocratic oath: "Whatever houses I may visit, I will come for the benefit of the sick, remaining free of all intentional injustice, of all mischief and in particular of sexual relations with both male and female, be they free or slaves."

Though medical school graduates today still swear to uphold the Hippocratic oath, when it comes to honoring the oath they face difficulties that are peculiar to our times. For more than two decades the delivery of health care in the U.S. has been jolted, upended and compromised by conflicting attitudes, policies and decisions, all aimed at shaping health care into a fiscally self-sustaining industry. Our nation's basic healthcare tenets have been challenged by managed care and government—determined policies creating new, painful dilemmas. The work of each individual physician is increasingly dictated by government policies, insurance payers and sometimes the medical establishment under whose auspices he or she aspires to deliver care. As rationing and ageism take root in our health care system, more and more people are falling into the ever-widening chasm between affordability and access to care.

The finite nature of health care resources demands that many suffer delayed or outright denial of medical treatment. Though the ostensible intent of rationing is the just allocation of these limited health care resources, the criteria that might compromise the ethics of fairness is like a tangled ball of yarn. Money plays a key role. The treatment a doctor considers both medically and ethically best for a patient may not be authorized by the entity that pays—an insurance company, Medicare or Medicaid.

The question of how to fairly allocate a limited resource is not new. George Bernard Shaw, the English playwright and author, probed the ethics of health care delivery and rationing in his play *The Doctor's Dilemma*, first staged in 1906. Though the play provided neither an answer nor a mechanism for rationing health care, nearly a century later Harvard Medical School clinical psychology professor Dr. James Sabin looked to Shaw as he wrestled with our current rationing challenge. Dr. Sabin felt that Shaw might comment today, "Anyone who looks in the Harvard Square doorways on a cold winter night and claims rationing doesn't exist is a fool. You are rationing health care every day—you can't avoid it. Figure out how to do it fairly."

How does one begin to allocate health care equitably? Until this century, Western societies regulated health care "naturally" with supply and demand. Wealth guaranteed certain people access to doctors, medicines, anesthesia and hospital beds. Those with money were sure to find a plentiful supply of the health care services they demanded. Those in or near the poverty line were confronted with fewer services. Someone with no money might not receive health care at all. The clear-cut "rules" of a wealth-based rationing system serves the haves and neglects the have-nots.

As the nineteenth-century progressed, the cruelty of wealth-based health care rationing began to trouble affluent citizens who had some resources to help equalize the situation. Furthermore, by then, local government had begun to recognize that public health was the concern of the entire community. Thus, at the local level, caring, visionary and financially solvent individuals banded together to address the health care needs of the poor.

In Boston many citizens came forward to help fill local health care gaps. The Jewish doctors, nurses and entrepreneurs who founded Beth Israel Hospital marshaled their resources to take care of the indigent, the city's most vulnerable. The Methodists, who founded the Deaconess Hospital, considered health care an integral part of their ministry. Both institutions, partnering over many decades with Harvard Medical School, helped make the allocation of medical resources more equitable by ensuring high-quality care for all—even those unable to pay for it themselves.

The national change that began with Franklin Delano Roosevelt's Depression-era federal programs for the indigent ultimately impacted both Beth Israel and the Deaconess—both community-based, service-driven health care providers—and forced them to reincarnate as a merged corporate entity focused intently on fiscal performance. History lauds FDR's New Deal for embracing our collective social responsibility to meet the basic needs of each citizen. Yet since the 1930s the government's role in apportioning health care has grown exponentially. From the Medicaid plan to aid U.S. elders to plans for universal health coverage each government "gift" to health care-seekers has come wrapped in mandates and controls that specify boiler-plate solutions to people's health care problems.

It does seem logical for the government to draw lines around what it will pay for. Elected officials court taxpayers' positive opinions and all policy-makers should aspire to cost-effective spending. However, each new restriction etched into the health care system removes choices from both patients and the doctors who deliver their care. Today, federal and state mandates guide—and sometimes supersede—your doctor in determining how your ills will be treated .The government seems to have no better idea how to apportion health care than a toddler trying to read James Joyce in Sanskrit.

Government mandates for health care delivery push uncomfortable rationing decisions all the way down the line in the system so that even the physician who is responsible by oath to focus on patient needs must wrestle with economics and ethics far outside his or her area of expertise. Today, every doctor must develop those areas of expertise. Dr. Mitchell Rabkin, president and CEO of Beth Israel Hospital before and shortly after its merger with Deaconess Hospital, learned this lesson the hard way. With his background as a physician and his long decades of service in administration of Beth Israel, Dr. Rabkin personified the caring doctor leading a caring institution.

In 1994 Beth Israel Hospital was on the fiscal brink—caught, like others, in the squeeze between rising costs and tightening controls by government and insurance payers—and was about to make a life-saving merger with Deaconess Hospital. Simultaneously, a federal task force on healthcare, led by First Lady Hillary Clinton, invited Dr. Rabkin to lend his name and share his thoughts about their well-publicized push for universal health care in the U.S.

Naturally, Dr. Rabkin accepted the invitation—after all, the notion of universal health care was in perfect tune with all Beth Israel stood for—and Beth Israel's public relations department issued a press release. Addressing the task force, Dr. Rabkin expressed enthusiasm for the concept of universal healthcare and noted, "With universal coverage no one is rationed out of the system."

Ironically for Dr. Rabkin, the federal bumbling toward a universal health care plan generated, in the short-term, more restrictive policies and spending caps that increased the rationing responsibilities that his administrative colleagues had left to him, his nurses and the staff physicians affiliated with Beth Israel Deaconess Medical Center. Since 1994, the trends have continued—higher medical expenses and spending caps that translate into rationing.

Beth Israel and Deaconess merged into a large, bottom-line-driven entity and Dr. Rabkin struggled to ensure consistent delivery of top-quality medical care. He faced external pressure from competitive institutions, an ongoing array of Beth Israel versus Deaconess culture clashes among doctors, nurses and other BIDMC staff, and increasing interference by government and insurance payers in the hospital's daily service to patients.

In Boston and elsewhere, inequities in health care access still exist and may even be increasing, with at least forty-five million citizens underinsured. Federal rules for health care allocation, combined with economic forces and demographic shifts, place intense fiscal pressure on every healthcare provider. In the past two decades, many medical practices and hospitals, traditionally those most responsive to the needs of people in their communities, have closed their doors. The disappearance of one's local hospital or doctor's office is a fierce form of rationing.

At its best-intentioned, rationing aims for equitable allocation of a limited resource. Yet in the end someone bears the burden of declaring that one person's life or quality of life matters more than someone else's. Policies, not people, appear to make decisions as to who shall live and who shall die.

The language of today's medical system beclouds the problem further by referring to patients as "units"—a dehumanizing term—or "consumers," which suggests a populace with full pockets and many options. Indeed, although all men and women are said to be created equal when it comes to health care access, some are still more equal than others. The affluent, educated and sophisticated "consumer" has a better chance than an indigent "unit" to receive the medical care he or she desires. Poorer, more marginalized people have fewer choices and are less apt to wend their way through a densely complicated health care system to obtain the care they require. The ideal of universal coverage seeks to equalize access for rich and poor, young and old, employed and unemployed. However, the realization of that ideal has proven to be elusive if not impossible.

Dr. Ben Gurian, a geriatric psychiatrist, delivered a sermon at the Arlington Street Church in Boston. He said, "The elderly American is a member of one of our most disenfranchised minority groups. Professional and non-professionals alike who are concerned with the aged population have a special obligation to speak on their behalf. The elderly are virtually without a voice in this highly competitive system where vested groups vie for a position in the national priorities.

"Our society has viewed the value of the senior citizen as decreasing with age so that it has been unwilling to spend what it considers inordinate amounts of money or services to provide for the maintenance of the elderly. It is not necessary that we passively accept the attitudes and conditions which currently exist. We have the opportunity to take appropriate action to help bring about fundamental change."

Dr. Gurian ended his sermon with a quote from John F. Kennedy: "It is not enough to add more years to our lives. We must add more life to our years." Dr. Gurian's sermon might well have been given this year. Actually, he presented it in 1971.

Many people are troubled by our system's failure to provide adequate health care for all. Yet, it is hard to imagine a community-based solution today. Federal rules for health care allocation, combined with economic forces and demographic shifts, place intense fiscal pressure on every health care provider. In the past two decades, many medical practices and hospitals have merged to take advantage of economies of scale while many smaller practices and hospitals—traditionally those most responsive to the needs of people in their communities—have closed their doors.

Internationally, healthcare rationing has been implemented in various forms and accordingly has been much discussed and debated. The first step is to acknowledge that as a limited resource, healthcare must somehow be rationed, as George Bernard Shaw recognized at the turn of the nineteenth century. In 1956, the British Royal Commission concluded that funding limitations would lead to a lack of care for patients who needed it. The British National Health Service left rationing to the discretion of physicians rather than specify its terms in public policy.

Canada's universal healthcare system today features price controls, virtually eliminating wealth as a criterion for obtaining care. Theoretically, the Canadian Health Care Act gives everyone access to every approved procedure .However, waiting lists for the most expensive procedures and the highest-priced, best-qualified doctors help to accomplish the rationing. Currently, in Canada, coronary bypass surgery has a thirty-week delay and indeed some patients may die while awaiting surgery. Even with the universal health care ideal driving its national and provincial policies,

Canada must creatively ration; a recent savings and restructuring plan in the province of Ontario eliminated some previously covered services for the elderly.

In Britain and Canada, where health care is theoretically free, people are deterred from obtaining health care by other costs; an enormous amount of self-rationing occurs. Sometimes, when the cost of medical care is too high, people even self-medicate with nonprescription drugs rather than seek the legitimate help that they need. Others are deterred from going to the doctor's office when they feel ill because of long waiting times for an appointment, the cost of time, travel, loss of wages and other issues. If everyone who purchased nonprescription drugs were to see a physician instead, the United States would require twenty-five times the current number of doctors. A more fair system would not force people to compare the value of health care with the financial, emotional or logistical cost of receiving it.

Many Western societies engage in bureaucratic rationing, which favors the patient who can self-advocate his or her way to the front of the line. The sophisticated, affluent or socially powerful almost always find their way to the care they require. Studies have shown that when transplants are rationed, bureaucracies appear to discriminate on the basis of income, race and sex, in that order. For example, a study by the Urban Institute found that for black and white males, the higher their income, the more likely they were to receive an organ transplant.

In the U.S., perhaps the most significant losses in medical care come from physicians' growing responsibility to participate in rationing. Sadly, today, many patients find themselves in adversarial relationships with their physicians at times when they most need to trust their medical caregivers.

When an acutely worried or critically ill patient needs care and may even have researched the treatment options, his or her doctor is the gatekeeper who may say, "No." The doctor may have many reasons for doing so. For one, he or she must "ration" his or her own time spent providing medical services. Most often a doctor's personal rationing follows the rules of common sense: "I will take only as many patients as I can competently care for."

Further, patients may not know the full cost of their treatment or understand how the system works—in particular that the cost of their treatment is borne by all members of their insurance plan or the medical practice. These financial concerns never leave the minds of today's doctors.

Another issue on doctors' minds, and likely the least of an ill patient's concern, is whether the patient's expected improvement in quality of life justifies an expensive medical intervention. According to some studies, physicians prioritize the patient's quality of life much less than patients do as a criterion for access to treatment.

Physician, economist and bio-ethicist Dr. Peter A. Ubel thinks that the debate should move forward from *whether* to ration health care to *how* to do so. Writing in the *Annals of Medicine*, Dr. Ubel lauds the Swedish Ministry of Health and Social Affairs for accepting rationing as inevitable. The Ministry's Health Care and Medical Priorities Commission took on the task of determining ethical values and principles—a map of priorities—that the national government could use to spark debate and inform decisions about how to ration health care. The commission's public officials, physicians, hospital administrators and professors held hearings with health care providers to study the conflict between need and resources.

The commission identified three core ethical precepts that must be applied to any plan for prioritizing health care delivery: individual autonomy, beneficence and justice. Autonomy implies patient choices and informed decision-making. Beneficence requires health professionals to respect and show consideration for the patient as a person while also considering the limited resources of the system. Justice requires that health care benefits be fairly distributed.

The commission stated that all human beings are equally valuable and that society must pay special attention to the needs of the weakest and most vulnerable, as well as to cost-efficiency. As paraphrased by Dr. Ubel, "Priorities should be set such that everyone is treated as a moral equal and there is to be no selecting-out of any vulnerable or frail group." All individuals should be provided equal opportunities to receive medical services regardless of race, ethnic group or gender.

The Swedish government now takes the lead in setting explicit health care priorities. They can enforce tax policies and impose mandates on medical training and research to assure that the priorities are followed. At the same time, Dr. Ubel asserts that physicians will always play a role in rationing and therefore should, as part of their standard medical training, acquire "the expertise to decide when to withhold health care from patients."

Talking about health care access in terms of priority-setting and acknowledging the moral content of rationing's difficult choices seems to have propelled the Swedish further down the road to health care reform than Hillary Clinton got by avoiding any talk of rationing at all.

Dr. Ubel believes that a year of life is worth $150,000 to $200,000 and suggests that the medical profession consider emotional factors as well when calculating cost. However, who should decide for the entire society what perspective to take and what valuation to set on emotional factors? For example, would everyone agree that we should provide all possible available care to veterans because they have defended our country? Should doctors use greater resources to palliate a terminally ill fifteen-year-old or a terminally ill seventy-five-year-old? Such decisions, no matter who makes them, ultimately represent the values of a nation or society. If we give primacy to preserving the lives of the young rather than the aged, we declare that elders' lives have less value.

Discussion of rationing often becomes contentious—and with good reason. Each of us has a personal, self-interested health care agenda as well as an emotional investment in the continued access to the care of our loved ones. We each view health care policies and realities through our own narrow prisms. Certain indignities and injustices may trouble us more than others.

In 1999, *The Boston Globe* reported public outrage over the state of Massachusetts' refusal to pay for a liver and lung transplant for an eighteen-year-old with cystic fibrosis. Individually, each organ to be transplanted was covered by insurance but the combined surgery was not on the approved list. The double procedure had never been done and thus had no proven results.

Public fundraising provided $250,000 to cover the cost of the surgery. Unfortunately, the patient died before two healthy organs were simultaneously available to complete the procedure.

Expensive procedures and treatments that help only a very few people create another level of quandary. Medical research that seeks new means of prolonging human life is very expensive. Each discovery yields new expensive treatments. In this world of health care rationing are medical advances a luxury we can afford? While important to those suffering from a particular condition or intrigued by the science behind a particular disease, medical research consumes dollars that could, for example, provide nebulizers for asthmatic inner-city children or prenatal care for impoverished pregnant women.

Further, more research has developed many marvelous treatments that are then rationed or priced out of the grasp of many who need them. For example, two decades of HIV/AIDS research has created effective treatments to protect the health of HIV-positive people—a benefit to those who have contracted HIV as well as to the societies and communities whose infection risk and cost of care for the terminally ill would be reduced by the treatments. However, many HIV-positive individuals both in the U.S. and abroad continue to lack access to these treatments.

A group of doctors and medical ethicists, including physicians from Brown and Harvard Universities, met in 2004 to develop national guidelines for rationing expensive, intensive-care treatments. Their motivations included cost control at a time when intensive-care hospital beds accounted for twenty percent of all hospital costs or $142 billion. In a *Boston Globe* article the physicians acknowledged their own practice of withholding treatment from the patients who would benefit the least.

Oregon, a medically sophisticated state, has concerns about cost effectiveness and yet assisted suicide is among the topics they will consider. They created a list of medical conditions that ranked treatment according to its projected effectiveness and cost/benefit. Preventive care such as mammograms topped the list while treatments for incurable ailments ranging from the common cold to end-stage cancer were at the bottom. About 700 medical problems are on the list and Oregon pays to treat about 550 of them.

How are their decisions made? "Likelihood of medical benefit" is often the primary criteria for allowing a patient access to a particular service. Some define "medical benefit" as a cure while others may accept prolonged life as a beneficial outcome. The next question is, "How long?" Some may try to evaluate the patient's anticipated contributions to society if his or her life is to be saved.

They are likely to base their evaluation on the patient's social status, education level and achievements in life thus far.

A typical benchmark is the patient's age: The older the patient, the less benefit assigned to the extension of his or her life. In countries that include the entire population in a single, government-funded health care plan, the elderly are usually pushed to the end of the rationing lines. Britain has a single-payer government health plan yet it is extremely difficult for an elderly patient to receive kidney dialysis or an organ transplant.

The medical director of a Texas hospital said that many procedures and medications are prohibited when it comes to the elderly. They only make exceptions for cases that provide unique opportunities for teaching medical students. In other words, an elderly patient may receive needed treatment if others—strangers—receive a tangible, useful benefit as well.

Age-based rationing policies find their logic in money. The U.S. population, overall, is aging. The elderly are the largest consumers of health care dollars. Women live longer than men and may have financially contributed less than their male counterparts. Should that be the determinant in their being rationed out of expensive health care? The percentage of the U.S. population over age sixty-five is nearly 12.5 percent (4.2 million) and is projected to increase. Particularly fast-growing are the ranks of the oldest old—people eighty years or above.

When a person's age becomes a key factor in limiting care, that disturbingly suggests that society has entirely abandoned the concept of fairness in rationing. A woman in her late seventies can be told that she may no longer receive physical therapy because her age yields a negative cost/benefit analysis. Is this fair? An elderly man can be denied cardiac surgery because he refuses to stop smoking and probably has, at most, a year to live. Is that fair? To apply calendar age as the primary determinant for services a patient may receive when approaching the end of life is indefensible. Age-based rationing equates being old with being moribund and denies the elderly equal consideration as persons of value in our society.

The Medicare system, launched in the U.S. in 1965, established a moral value and a national goal of ensuring health care to the nation's elders. It covers all patients who are over sixty-two or disabled for both inpatient and outpatient services. Poverty in the elderly population decreased after Medicare eliminated its recipients' out-of-pocket medical care expenses.

Medicaid, a separate government plan, was designed to cover the underinsured and uninsured by reimbursing physicians and hospitals at least partially for the market value of their services. Today, however, providing Medicaid services at delayed and low reimbursement rates increases the fiscal pressure on a physician's practice or a hospital—it simply costs too much.

Many elderly recipients of Medicare and Medicaid can barely manage to scrape together the money to purchase prescribed medications and food at the same time. When an elderly person chooses food and sacrifices medication, a particularly brutal form of health care rationing takes place.

Proponents of age-based health care rationing warn that society cannot bear the economic strain that will follow the retirement of the baby boomer generation. Dr. Daniel Callahan, co-founder the Hastings Center, writes in *Setting Limits: Medical Goals in an Aging Society,* "…medicine should not be used for the further extension of life of the aged but only for the full achievement of a natural and fitting life span and/or the relief of suffering." This philosophy would allow the Medicare and Medicaid system to use an age-based standard to restrict coverage for life-extending treatment such as organ transplants, cardiac bypass surgery and kidney dialysis. With huge gaps in medical coverage in the United States and the baby boomers headed for retirement, the consideration of age-based rationing is even more critical today than it has ever been.

Dr. Callahan sees age-based rationing as a necessary response to health care's financial problems: "There may be no limits on how far we can go, but there are limits of what we can pay for." He notes that the fastest-growing age group, eighty and older, is the very population that requires expensive and intensive medical care. Plagued by chronic illnesses, many elderly occupy hospital beds longer and use more of their doctors' time than younger patients. Indeed, it is estimated that the government now spends more than $9,000 per elderly person and less than $900 per child each year. Thus some proponents of age-based rationing see it as a way to restore justice while saving money.

Dr. Callahan has proposed that the government refuse to pay for life-extending medical care for individuals beyond the age of seventy or eighty and only pay for palliative, pain-relieving treatment. He argues that a patient's need should not be "a fundamental criterion for determining how much health care the elderly [patient] is allotted." He further states that in the context of constant technological innovations that prolong life, the "needs of the elderly know no bounds and drain the pool of resources that ought to be made available to all age groups." He contends that by the age of seventy or eighty, a person has lived out a natural life span and achieved most of life's goals and possibilities and ought not receive treatments to "extend their lives at the expense of those who have not lived out a normal life span."

This arbitrary decision would not take into account older individuals who have made incredible contributions to society and indeed may continue to contribute even beyond a cut-off age if permitted, for example, to obtain dialysis three times a week. Should Sigmund Freud, at age eighty-three, have been denied treatment for throat cancer because he required expensive medication? John Kenneth Galbraith died at the age of ninety. He was an active and brilliant man who continued to contribute knowledge until one week before his death, when he was scheduled to speak at Harvard's Kennedy School of Government (unfortunately, he was unable to deliver it). Before Eleanor Roosevelt's death at seventy-eight she was still able to drive herself from New York to Maine; her value to our country was incalculable. Grandma Moses was still painting at age 101.

Unanticipated, extenuating individual circumstances that arise in the case of each patient must be considered: No two dilemmas are exactly the same, particularly at the end of life. When a patient is sustained on artificial life support with no expectation of recovery, should we evaluate the worth of the comatose or brain-dead individual solely in terms of their cost of maintenance? Ariel Sharon has been on life support since 2006 with no expectation of recovery. Where do we factor in respect for his achievements and the value of his contributions to the world? Who will ultimately make and own the decision to remove the former Israeli leader's ventilator? Will cost or compassion pull the trigger?

The debate goes on. In an ideal system a terminally ill patient would have the choice of when and how to end his or her own life. In olden times the Eskimos placed their elderly on ice floes and pushed them out to sea. Rationing or choice? Some have suggested that we construct ways for patients to pay for their own end-of-life care through medical savings and reimbursements from insurers. How would the indigent, the uninformed and those of unsound mind participate in such a scheme? Would Medicaid pick up the slack to ensure these elders the same end-of-life options as their more financially resourceful peers?

Some say that rationing by age is acceptable if there is no better alternative. Hard-line critics of Dr. Callahan say that his ideas are ageist, classist and sexist. Women tend to live longer than men, after all, and under his rationing scheme more women would be denied more care for a greater number of years. Many believe that a first-come, first-served or lottery system would be a more equitable and ethically justifiable way to allocate healthcare than using age as a primary criterion.

Even if financial savings were achieved by rationing care by age and new funds entered the government's coffers, there's no guarantee that any of those savings would improve the overall health of our citizenry or be allocated to health care at all. Any health care savings achieved by a rationing plan—or any other way—may be subsumed by other national priorities. As determined by the last administration, one might be as likely to see savings redirected toward the continuingly costly war in Iraq or the demands of homeland security as toward the ever-escalating cost of medications and medical technology or meaningful steps toward universal health care.

Health care rationing is a reality as we struggle to balance the needs of a changing population against our limited supply of resources. Yet the right to health care should not diminish with age. In allocating healthcare, relevant factors ought to include the acuity of a patient's need, the likelihood of improving the quality of his or her life and the contributions that person has made to society.

The criteria we elect are important and should be considered carefully because they establish social precedents with implications that reach beyond the world of doctors and hospitals.

A later chapter of this book discusses the 1918 influenza pandemic and its impact on local health care delivery resources in Boston. For the past eighty-six years the government has made heroic efforts through pharmaceutical companies, the CDC, the FDA and the National Institutes of Health to provide the population with an influenza vaccine to avert a reoccurrence. The pharmaceutical companies produced a sufficient supply of vaccine, changing the formula each year to deflect the mutating virus.

Today there is escalating concern about a potential, new public health disaster: the swine flu. On the cusp of the 2004 election, President Bush abstained from commenting on the potential avian flu epidemic while his administration put out the word that healthy adults should forgo flu shots—a strategy more helpful to public budgets than to public health.

At the time, Dr. Marcia Angell, author of the 2004 expose *The Truth About the Drug Companies*, urged a different plan, suggesting that the government declare an emergency and purchase all available shots. To date no national plan has been announced. We as a nation would have been wise to think this through in advance.

Few if any of us recall the pandemic of 1918. Now, almost a century later, the unanticipated swine flu has felled a twenty-three-month-old Mexican child, echoing the 1918 influenza pandemic. The World Health Organization raised a Phase 5 immediate alert—the next-highest level in the global warning system. Within forty-eight hours of the first death, Dr. Margaret Chan, general director of the organization, said at a news conference in Geneva that all nations should be on high alert for "unusual outbreaks" of influenza or pneumonia. The Centers for Disease Control and Prevention reported ninety-one confirmed cases in ten states, sixty-four of which occurred in five states alone.

Dr. Chan emphasized the need for calm but spoke as if a pandemic had already begun, noting that the World Health Organization was tracking the "pandemic." She also emphasized that developing countries tended to have more severe flu epidemics than "rich" ones, and that her organization and others would need to make special offers to help poorer nations.

President Obama took the unusual step of using a prime-time, televised news conference to mark his one-hundredth day in office and deliver his health message: He advised Americans to wash their hands, cover their mouths when they cough, stay home if they are sick and keep their children out of school for any illnesses. He also called on Congress to authorize $1.5 billion toward monitoring and tracking the swine flu virus as well as creating a supply of antiviral medications.

As more communities became affected by what is now known as the AH1N1 virus, the efforts of pubic health facilities became much more visible. Since the announcement of the first case on April 29, 2009 and as of this writing, there have been 642 cases confirmed in forty-one states, and over 400 in Mexico. The age range of the stricken is twenty-two months to eighty-one years. A public health emergency was announced and antiviral drugs are being stockpiled.

In an effort to protect the populace, the question of whether to close the borders was considered. However, if that were done, it would not only fail to stop the virus but would also cause economic collapse and possibly add to the death rate. Many necessary goods required during a pandemic come from overseas suppliers, thereby extending the length of time for delivery.

The swine flu virus seems to be susceptible to two prescription drugs: Tamiflu and Relenza, both of which can shorten the course of the illness. Dr. Ericson noted that we have stockpiles of such medications but if a real pandemic were to develop, we may use up all we have. It's been proposed that the vaccine should be given only to those who are seriously ill and hospitalized—those for whom it could be a matter of life or death.

Two very different current trends in health care delivery bear mentioning in the context of rationing. First, the introduction of a new medical professional: the hospitalist, a term coined by Dr. Robert M. Wachter and Dr. Lee Goldman in 1996. A hospitalist is a physician employed by a hospital as a main provider and coordinator of care for inpatients who are admitted through the emergency room and are without a primary care physician. In short, the hospitalist is the patient's primary care physician for the duration of the hospital stay. Generally, hospitalists are empowered to coordinate

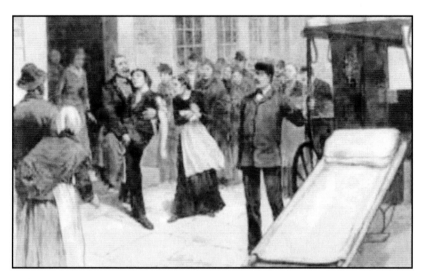

Influenza pandemic.

patient care, order tests and make treatment decisions in consultation with primary care physicians. They are trained to respond quickly to changes in a patient's condition.

A study by the National Association of Inpatient Physicians reported that about fifty percent of hospitalists were trained as general medical internists and forty percent as medical subspecialists. The hospitalist model seeks to enhance the quality and efficiency of inpatient care. In recent years, the model has enjoyed widespread acceptance by both physicians and hospital administrators who recognize the need for the hospitalist's presence; they find that it benefits patients, shows positive medical outcomes and increases efficiency.

With hospitals ever-mindful of costs, a study from the University of Chicago Hospital reported reductions in overall costs and short-term mortality with the introduction of the hospitalist model. Many primary care physicians hope the adoption of the new specialty will decrease their job stress and improve their lifestyles, as they will no longer be required to follow their surgical or acutely ill patients into the hospital environment. Some medical staff members think that the hospitalists help solve the long-standing problem of finding physicians to care for patients admitted from an emergency department who have no primary care provider.

On the down side, there are concerns that a transitory primary care relationship interrupts a patient's continuity of care. For example, as medical charts pass through several pairs of hands, information may get lost. In addition, some patients may not accept the new model of care. Still, occupancy of hospital beds is increasing as the population ages; thus, hospitalists are likely to be in greater demand to provide care during longer hospital stays.

Hospitalists represent the fastest-growing field in medicine, according to the press and hospital administrators. The BIDMC was one of the first Boston-area hospitals to offer this service and hospitalists now care for about sixty percent of BIDMC's general medical admissions. Recently, Mt. Auburn Hospital in Cambridge, Massachusetts, a member of CareGroup, tripled their number of hospitalists as well.

While hospitals aim to streamline and improve inpatient care with hospitalists, a new and completely different health care delivery system has sprung up outside hospital walls: boutique or concierge medicine, a trend that works at the other end of the spectrum. These medical practices create a supply-and-demand market for medical care in which wealthy patients and their physicians elect to participate in virtually independent of the restrictive overall health care system. Vigorously debated by the medical establishment and healthcare consumers, the boutique system serves those who can pay a large amount of money upfront.

Dr. Flier, a senior physician at Beth Israel, launched this new, private delivery of medical care in Boston. Formerly a senior physician at Beth Israel, he served as vice chairman for research and was a member of Dr. Robert Meltzer's turnaround team to improve BIDMC in 2001. In a *Boston Globe* interview, he said, "My feelings are deep and strong about this institution [BIDMC] but we'd better change things."

Shortly thereafter, he gathered a handpicked group of physicians and patients to form a boutique/concierge practice. Several hundred people were invited to pay an annual retainer of several thousand dollars to receive their medical care from the group. As more boutique practices came on the scene, each practice determined its annual retainer.

According to an article in *The New York Times* by Amy Zitkin, annual retainers for boutique health care in Florida and Seattle can reach $20,000. One Florida-based boutique group, MDVIP, serves patients throughout the U.S. and advertises in local newspapers and on television with commercials featuring local doctors.

Group members can reach their doctor at any hour, day or night, by cell phone if necessary. When they visit their physician, patients find a waiting room that is quiet and tastefully furnished. Their doctor will accompany the patient to a specialist if warranted. A "super" annual examination is provided and they offer same-day or next-day appointments. There are no constraints on the amount of time the physician spends with the patient.

Some view boutique medicine as the wealthy feeling deservedly entitled while others—the boutiques' patients—find it to be the best thing that could have happened to them. This mode of delivering health care probably strays far from most physicians' original intent upon graduation from medical school. However, medical practice and health care delivery in the United States have become so convoluted, they're barely recognizable when compared to the 1950s model, before extensive government interference set in.

The medical boutique may represent some doctors' response to a bundle of professional frustrations including ever-rising malpractice insurance costs, a litigious society, towers of paper work, reduced reimbursements from insurance companies and feelings of regret that must surely result from seeing too many patients for too brief a visit each day.

Chapter Two

In the Beginning

"Whoever saves a single life, it is as if he saved the world."
—The Talmud

The city of Boston was founded on September 17, 1630, on a peninsula surrounded by the waters of Massachusetts Bay. The colonists had first encamped at what is now Charlestown. However, the site lacked potable water, necessitating their relocating to today's Beacon Hill, which offered a freshwater spring close to the natural harbor. The intersection of State and Washington streets, now Boston's financial district, was the early settlement's center.

The Native American inhabitants, the Algonquins, whom the colonists displaced, named the area "Shawmut" and later changed the name to Boston. Over the years, the populace gave the city its enduring nicknames. During the Revolutionary War, Boston was known as "the Cradle of Liberty." The Reverend John Winthrop, first governor of Massachusetts, created the name "City on the

Hill" in a Sunday sermon. Some referred to Boston as "Beantown," honoring the popular, local delicacy of baked beans made with molasses imported from the Caribbean. Justice Oliver Wendell Holmes dubbed Boston "The Hub of the Universe" and is said to have coined the term "Brahmin" for the Boston aristocracy—the Yankee families that controlled much of Boston's wealth and power.

The early Anglo-Saxon settlers were an educated group who lived within a strictly structured society and followed a rigid work ethic. Early on they created institutions that established education and medicine as bedrocks of their society. Boston Latin School, established in 1635, is to this day a highly respected public secondary school. The following year, Harvard University was founded—the first university in the United States.

Boston flourished as a prime intellectual and cultural center and, with industrialization, developed and thrived as a center of commerce. Ships docked daily in the city's large and welcoming harbor, bringing goods and people. Thousands of Irish immigrants arrived, fleeing the potato famine. Eager to work, they had marshaled their courage to transform their grim lives of persecution or starvation. Jewish immigrants fleeing *pogroms* came from Central Europe and later from Eastern Europe—Russia, Hungary, Latvia and Romania. The immigrants crowded into existing neighborhoods along the waterfront: the North End and Fort Hill areas.

This rapid increase in population presented many problems, though the immigrants were welcomed as a source of low-cost labor. Usually, they arrived impoverished with neither relatives to help them adjust to the new city nor employment opportunities awaiting them. They also faced major difficulties in assimilation. Lacking knowledge of the city or language, they struggled to find jobs. The Irish immigrants came from agrarian rather than industrialized societies and were ill-prepared to work in Boston's burgeoning industry and commerce.

By 1909 about 80,000 Jews had gathered in the north and west ends of Boston. Their neighborhoods became known as the Jewish ghettos. The North End was a triangular plot of land, each leg measuring one quarter of a mile. The West End covered comparable acreage. In both neighborhoods, new arrivals found deplorable housing conditions. They crowded into filthy, unventilated, vermin-infested tenements, and disease was all too readily transmitted from resident to resident.

All immigrants arrived requiring medical care. By the dawn of the twentieth century, the medical care they needed, theoretically, could be found in Boston—a city rich with hospitals. The Boston Dispensary was founded in 1796, Massachusetts General in 1811 and Boston Lying-In, the city's first maternity hospital, in 1832. The Free Hospital for Women opened in 1875, Mt. Auburn Hospital in 1871 in Cambridge, Children's Hospital in 1869, Peter Bent Brigham in 1913 and Massachusetts Eye and Ear in 1827. However, this array of institutions primarily provided care to Anglo-Saxons and resisted or outright refused to treat Jews and the Irish. Massachusetts General hospital claimed, "The admission of such patients creates in the minds of our citizens a prejudice against the hospital making them unwilling to enter it and thus tends to directly lower the general standing and character of its inmates." Admitting physicians were advised to "use utmost vigilance to avoid admitting them." Consequently, a large population remained underserved.

Jewish immigrants rarely sought help from gentile charities, doubtless feeling a lingering mistrust of the gentiles who had oppressed them in Europe. Another obstacle to obtaining medical care was the immigrants' adherence to Orthodox Jewish rituals and dietary restrictions. Perhaps their greatest limitation was language. Many Jewish immigrants arrived unable to speak or understand English, making it difficult for members of the medical community to provide them with care. Boston's physicians had as little knowledge of Yiddish and Hebrew as they did of Jewish culture, social mores, religious traditions and rules for strict observance of the Sabbath.

Dr. Richard Clarke Cabot, professor of social ethics at Harvard Medical School and a senior practicing physician at Massachusetts General Hospital, ordered a study of patients who showed evidence of "Hebraic debility." Recognizing that Jewish patients were not receiving care comparable to that of MGH's gentile patients and noting some symptoms that seemed peculiar to the Jewish patients, Dr. Cabot assigned Dr. Hyman Morrison, a Harvard medical student at MGH, to "study these patients, visiting them in their homes, so as to get details of their ailments and observe their modes of living." In 1907, Dr. Morrison published his observations, stating that "the prevalent patient's symptoms are pain, constipation, and apprehension" and "the etiology of these debilitating conditions is to be traced to the peculiar circumstances under which Jews lived, and still live, here in America. The economic strain during the early years after arrival is another important factor." The study further noted that Jewish patients' "complaints had been generally misunderstood because they couldn't explain their pain" in English, creating a language barrier.

Dr. Cabot reasoned that Jewish physicians could better understand and treat these patients. Unfortunately, practicing Jewish physicians in Boston were few. In 1898 only thirty-six of Boston's 1,550 physicians were Jewish. Most were European-born and had received medical degrees in their homelands; very few had graduated from American schools. The fourteen most active Jewish doctors practicing in Boston's West End were all under the age of thirty-four.

Existing Boston medical schools operated on a quota system, which allowed for the admission of very few Jewish medical students. In Waltham, Massachusetts, where Brandeis University now stands, the mediocre Middlesex Medical School accepted Jewish applicants. Though licensed to practice, it was rare for them to acquire staff privileges at the Boston hospitals. Thus, in those early days, a Jewish doctor saw his patients in their overcrowded homes or in a makeshift office within his own home. At a time when people traveled by horse, on foot or by horse-drawn buggy, arranging a doctor's visit was confusing and costly for patients. Caring for an impoverished clientele was tiring and time-consuming for doctors. The health problems of the immigrant population were exacerbated by miserable living conditions in Boston's Jewish ghettoes and the residents' inability to afford adequate nourishment.

Members of two religious denominations—Methodist and Jewish—were appalled that so many hundreds of people lacked adequate medical care. Their independent efforts to mitigate the situation led to the founding of two hospitals, each destined for renown and longevity: New England Deaconess and Beth Israel. Nearly 100 years later, in 1996, both institutions once again confronted a crisis in health care delivery. Motivated by the mutual need to maintain fiscal solvency and continue to deliver high-quality health care, the Beth Israel and Deaconess hospitals undertook a difficult though ultimately successful merger. In this chapter, we explore the roots of each institution's particular mission and culture so we may better understand why and how the hospitals joined

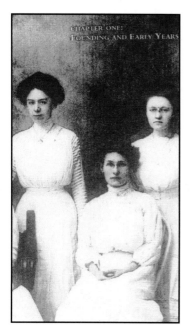

together to pursue their basic purpose of providing compassionate, exemplary health care for both the underserved and the financially solvent.

Ultimately, the single, shared mission was the saving grace that made Beth Israel Deaconess Medical Center (BIDMC) possible. Despite the differences in philosophies, personalities and underpinnings that comprised each hospital, both hospitals focused on providing the best possible medical care. Both institutions built their success on policies that nurtured loyal employees. A for-

Deaconess nurses.

mer Deaconess administrator (now emeritus), Richard Lee, described the hospital's long-standing philosophy: "If you want people to take good care of patients, take care of people"—a philosophy espoused independently, almost word for word, by the Beth Israel Hospital staff and trustees interviewed in 2003.

The Deaconess Order of the Methodist Church dates back to 1836 Germany, where a Lutheran pastor, Reverend Theodor Fleidler, and his wife, Frederika, established a small facility for discharged prisoners. Over time, the facility expanded to include an orphanage, a training school and a small hospital. The school taught all elements of nursing care and was open only to unmarried women. Some became deaconesses on completion of their training. One of the Fleidlers' students in mid-nineteenth-century Germany was British-born Florence Nightingale, who became legendary for ministering to the wounded on Europe's battlefields. The word "deaconess" derives from Greek and means servant, clergy, patroness, abbess and priestess. From its beginnings in Europe, the Deaconess movement became part of the Methodist Church in America.

In April 1886, the New England Conference of Methodists recognized the need to provide health care services for the region's many immigrant and indigent families, whose abject poverty and ignorance of social customs prevented them from properly caring for themselves. Like the immigrant Jews, this broader population knew little about how to access medical care. In 1889 the New England Home and Training School bought a five-story brownstone

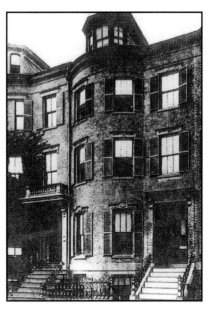

The first inpatient Deaconess Hospital.

at 691 Massachusetts Avenue in Boston and created a fourteen-bed hospital.

Mary E. Lunn, a deaconess from Chicago, was appointed the

first superintendent of the Deaconess Hospital in 1897, located on Massachusetts Avenue in Boston. She had trained as a nurse in Chicago and fulfilled the additional criteria for the senior position. A deaconess had to be between twenty-three and forty years of age and required not only a certificate of good health from her own doctor but a recommendation from her pastor as well. Ten women staffed the new hospital: Deaconess Mary Lunn, several deaconess candidates and independent physicians. The hospital was founded to meet a human need with the recognition that, as Deaconess Lunn wrote, "Science and kindliness should unite to combat disease."

Deaconesses were trained to be nurses, not physicians, and in the early years their work was missionary. Their primary task was to provide religious counseling to critically ill patients in their homes. The Methodists deployed a deaconess to assuage spiritual and moral as well as physical ills. A Deaconess noted, "One frequently meets people upon the streets, especially in those crowded and poverty-stricken districts, where sin, suffering, and sickness prevail." With that in mind, "The duties of the deaconess are to minister to the poor, visit the sick, pray with the dying, care for the orphans, seek the wandering, comfort the sorrowing, and save the sinners."

While each deaconess readily accepted these major demands, the truly burdensome requirement may have been to relinquish all other pursuits. A deaconess wore a black or gray habit and worked without pay. In 1929 deaconesses abandoned the habit for contemporary clothing and began receiving salaries and pension benefits as befitted professionally trained workers. Now they enjoyed the freedom to marry and have children. However, they had to remain committed to a life of service and discipline, and to the community. In addition, the position of president shifted from a deaconess to a male physician or businessman. Deaconesses then focused solely on teaching in the hospital's school of nursing.

From the outset, the founders of the New England Deaconess hospital sought to create a home-like atmosphere. Financially solvent patients preferred to be treated in their own homes by nurses or caretakers, and doctors made house calls. Indigent patients

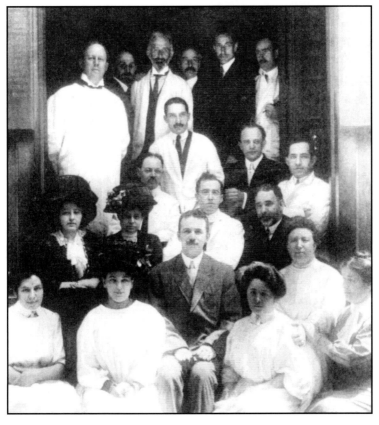

Deaconesses and physicians.

were treated in the hospital. The Deaconess administration, board of trustees and medical staff all agreed that the hospital would specialize in specific areas of medicine and surgery rather than become a full-service general hospital. The plan reflected the rapid refinement and growing popularity of surgery.

In 1896 the Deaconess Hospital on Massachusetts Avenue opened with surgery as its primary service. The hospital attracted a salaried staff of leading medical practitioners as well as a home base for neophyte physicians who were beginning their medical practices.

Among several pillars of the hospital, two were outstanding: Dr. Elliot Joslin and Dr. Frank Lahey. Dr. Joslin opened his first office in 1908 in his father's house in Boston. Though he began his career in the general practice of medicine, he soon became interested in diabetes and gradually narrowed his focus to metabolic research and the treatment of diabetic individuals. At that time the only known treatment for diabetes was to severely reduce food intake: Some patients died of poor nutrition and near-starvation. In 1921 two Canadian researchers developed insulin. The following year, Dr. Joslin became the first doctor in Boston to treat patients with insulin.

The significance of insulin treatment for diabetes was immediately recognized by the Massachusetts Department of Public Health. Initially, insulin was provided to doctors free of charge. Dr. Joslin's work was so successful, he soon became a world authority on the treatment of diabetes. The Joslin Clinic opened at Deaconess Hospital in 1952 and remains a prime research facility and center for treatment of diabetics.

At this same time, Dr. Frank Lahey, who considered himself a general surgeon, was actually specializing in the surgical treatment of goiters and the thyroid gland. Many of his patients also had cardiac problems. In 1920 he performed 168 thyroid operations, only three of which resulted in death of the patient—an unusual outcome for the time. His skills were considered remarkable. Born in Haverhill, Massachusetts, Dr. Lahey was a Harvard Medical School graduate who had trained as a surgeon at Boston City Hospital. He established one of the first group medical practices in 1923—the Lahey Clinic—which included a gastroenterologist, an anesthesiologist and a surgeon. Initially, his office was housed in an apartment on Beacon Street in Boston that had previously been his home. The clinic then affiliated with the Deaconess and New England Baptist hospitals and evolved into the internationally renowned Lahey Clinic.

While the Deaconess was evolving into medical specialties and surgery, less than a mile away, a similar but broader grassroots effort was in process among members of the Jewish community. Young, entrepreneurial businessmen were establishing themselves in Boston and had begun to accrue financial resources to aid their community. They were committed to addressing the medical needs of their underserved kinfolk. Guided by the Talmudic ideal that opened this chapter, these Jewish businessmen, along with doctors, rabbis and community leaders, founded the Mt. Sinai Association. They successfully created a medical facility for the poor of all races and ethnicities. Their mission was to create a Jewish hospital in Boston where service to others was fundamental and doctors of all religions could practice medicine, thereby meeting the needs of the underserved populations. Although their aim was to create a hospital for the Jews of Boston, the association stipulated from the beginning that they would not refuse any patient seeking care regardless of their creed, race or religion.

One of the Mt. Sinai Association's early leaders was Dr. Harry Linenthal, a Jewish immigrant who, by the turn of the century, had become a physician, an inspector of sanitation of clothing factories for the Massachusetts Department of Public Health, and a member of a state committee on health standards for working children. Born in 1876 in a small, Russian town, Harry had emigrated with his parents in 1891 and settled in Boston's West End. As a youth, he had worked days and studied English in the evening. After graduating with several honors from English High School in 1896, he'd became one of only two graduates in his class to go to Harvard College. He'd graduated *magna cum laude* and *cum laude* from Harvard Medical School in 1904.

Dr. Linenthal was the first Jewish physician appointed to the staff of the MGH, where he worked in the nerve clinic. His appointment was achieved by the intense lobbying of Dr. Richard Clarke Cabot, a senior physician at Massachusetts General Hospital. He told Dr. Linenthal he was "disturbed that the hospital [MGH] had gone 101 years without a single Jewish doctor on staff. Such exclusion had to be remedied." Their mutual involvement in the creation of the Mt. Sinai dispensaries demonstrated the commitment of both men to the establishment of a nondiscriminatory medical center in Boston.

The association's task was daunting and its progress slow. The group focused first on the financing, acquisition and reconstruction of the property that would become the first Mt. Sinai dispensary in August 1902. Two separate outpatient clinics—for men and women—occupied mirror-image sides of 105 Chambers

Street in downtown Boston, not far from the MGH. The original building has been described as a storefront and basement. The ground floor was divided into seven rooms: waiting room, apothecary and five clinic rooms for medical, eye, ear, nose and throat care in each dispensary. The founders recognized that they would have to compensate for their patients' language difficulties and so specified that prescription instructions and labels would be written in English and Yiddish.

In its first eight months of operation, 5,707 patients received care at the Mt. Sinai dispensary and by year's end, 10,000 patients had been treated. By 1904 Dr. Cabot had become increasingly concerned about the medical plight of the Jews he had been seeing at MGH. His involvement with Mt. Sinai and its staff grew even closer. He was impressed by the Mt. Sinai physicians, twenty of who had been his students at Harvard Medical School. According to Dr. Linenthal, Dr. Cabot praised the quality of their practice, noting their patience with those seeking care and their reluctance to overmedicate. A renowned teacher and a most successful physician, he also wrote prodigiously. He seemed to be watching over the dispensaries. Readily he offered suggestions to the Mt. Sinai staff, who were very receptive to his forward-thinking notions regarding dispensary practice.

Dr. Cabot became president of the Mt. Sinai medical staff in 1907 and remained in that position for seven years. Dr. Arthur Linenthal—the son of Dr. Harry Linenthal—raised the question in his book, *First a Dream*, "Why did Dr. Cabot, a Boston Brahmin, accept the presidency of the Mt. Sinai staff and bring his prestige to this small Jewish institution?" Though the question remains unanswered he was described as a man of conviction and vision with the ability to recognize and support valuable, credible, creative ideas. With deep moral convictions and boundless enthusiasm for teaching, Dr. Cabot suggested that nurses be employed to assist doctors in the clinics and to visit patients at home. When the tuberculosis epidemic began, he promptly formed a clinic.

The dispensaries required additional space to serve the growing number of patients arriving at their doors. Promptly, the association rented a second building within walking distance, at 17 Staniford Street. This four-story building provided seven rooms: two interior stairways, fifteen patient beds, an operating room, a kosher kitchen, a bedroom for nurses and a dining room. The staircases served as waiting rooms.

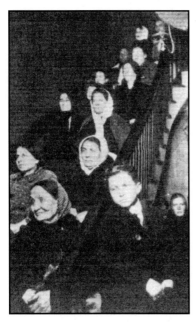

Without a waiting room, Mt. Sinai patients use the staircase.

During the years of the Mt. Sinai dispensaries on Chambers and Staniford streets, tuberculosis was spreading throughout the city of Boston. Lung damage and 1,300 tuberculosis-related deaths occurred in Boston in 1904. Across the Commonwealth of Massachusetts, local women banded together to form hands-on societies to provide help, including the Boston Association for the Relief and Control of Tuberculosis and the National Association for the Study and Prevention of Tuberculosis. Intense fear was engendered by the epidemic—particularly because of the threat to already-compromised, underserved immigrants who were living in squalor. The poverty and cramped quarters heightened their anxiety. The women in the Jewish community became actively involved in both the Mt. Sinai project and the battle against tuberculosis. In May 1910, they formed an auxiliary—Mt. Sinai Association—and charged one dollar a year for membership. Subsequently, the group grew to 350 members.

Meanwhile, many middle-class women volunteered to learn about the proper care of consumptives and contributed their time, funds and knowledge to help stricken families. The volunteers of the Jewish Women's Anti-Tuberculosis Association became actively engaged in patient care and support for families. They built an infrastructure that evolved into the first social service department in a Jewish hospital.

The Mt. Sinai Association's Women's Auxiliary met in one another's homes, in their synagogues and temples, planning fundraising activities to financially support the creation of the first Jewish inpatient hospital. Auxiliary women walked door to door from the West End of Boston to Brookline, climbing innumerable flights of tenement stairs, selling miniature bricks at five cents each. The auxiliary raised $5,000, which helped fund the purchase of the Dennison Estate, its extensive renovations and new medical and surgical equipment. They then presented an additional $150 check when the hospital opened.

The Women's Auxiliary has continued its fundraising efforts to the present day. For many decades, the group's events included black-tie balls, concerts, banquets and educational meetings; women's luncheons were regularly oversubscribed and all proceeds were donated to the Mt. Sinai Hospital—later to Beth Israel Hospital.

Donors' names were inscribed in the "Golden Book" and to this day the auxiliary presents a sizable check at the annual meeting of the Beth Israel Deaconess Medical Center.

Even more active on the front lines of the tuberculosis epidemic were fifty young, unmarried West End women who formed the Jewish Anti-Tuberculosis Association in 1907. Mt. Sinai dispensary nurse Mary Lurie recruited, organized and supervised the group with the motto "Make War on Consumption." The Jewish Anti-Tuberculosis Association and a Commonwealth of Massachusetts application was filed for incorporation as a charitable organization. Under the headline "Jewish Girls Fight the Plague," *The Boston Post* referred to the group as "one of the most remarkable organizations in Boston."

The group members were teenage girls whose working-class parents encouraged them to work for humanity. Physicians taught the young women about tuberculosis: the method of contagion, the symptoms and the effects on the economic lives of afflicted families and communities. With a deep understanding of the problems associated with tuberculosis, the girls of the Jewish Anti-Tuberculosis Association were each assigned particular sections of Boston to investigate the incidence of the disease. They visited their patients—Jewish and gentile—to make sure that each patient followed his or her prescribed regimen.

The knowledge physicians imparted to the girls of the Jewish Anti-Tuberculosis Association was based on the findings of Dr. Robert Koch, born December 11, 1843. In 1882, after many years of intensive investigation and experimentation, Dr. Koch reported that *tubercle bacillus* was the bacterium that caused consumption—then renamed "tuberculosis." In 1905 Dr. Koch was awarded the Nobel

Prize for physiology and medicine. He had shown positive proof that the disease was contagious and determined it could be prevented by breaking the cycle of person-to-person infection. For treatment he prescribed a rigorous, prolonged program of exposure to fresh air. Patients and families were urged to live outdoors all the time, rain or shine. His advice for afflicted city dwellers included a roof-top tent or an outdoor bedroom on a porch with an overhead cover.

To create an outdoor bed, doctors advised patients to use chairs with footstools. Ideally, Dr. Koch thought it best for patients to receive treatment away from their homes. His advice was immediately heeded and Massachusetts was the first state to build private and public sanatoria. Patients were admitted to Boston Consumptive Hospital in Mattapan in 1909.

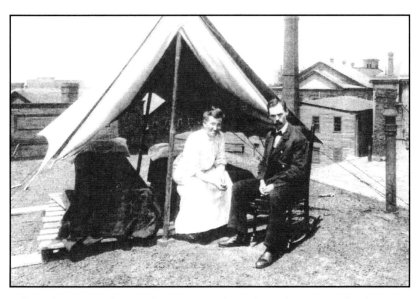

Tuberculin patients live outdoors. Picture from the Tufts-New England Medical Center.

The tubercular patient's diet consisted of three daily meals supplemented by two quarts of milk or eight to twelve eggs. Personal hygiene and regular hand washing were emphasized to prevent the spread of infection. Separate silverware and dishes were to be washed in boiling water; bed linens were to be boiled and then dried in the sun on the clotheslines. The patient's sputum was to be collected and burned.

Few medications were available or prescribed, other then heroin or codeine, for a cough that disturbed sleep. Nux vomica or gentian—a bitter digestive stimulant—might have been prescribed to ease stomach pain and stimulate appetite. Today, nux vomica is recommended for anorexia and atonic dyspepsia; it improves nourishment especially in the elderly.

Besides addressing the physical treatment and comfort of the affected patients, each girl talked with family members about contagion, helped arrange financial assistance when a wage-earner was too sick to work, and approached charitable organizations for financial support of the families. They solicited donations of household supplies such as sheets, cutlery, towels and blankets since the affected families could not afford these expenses. Their enthusiasm and consistent weekly visits brought a sense of hope and their pleasant demeanors encouraged the sick and their families. In short, the teenage volunteers of the Jewish Anti-Tuberculosis Association did much the same work that professional, credentialed social workers do today.

As some of these young women married, the organization bylaws were amended to allow them to remain members of the group. Junior groups were formed for young teenage women in 1911. The groups raised money through bazaars, amateur theatricals and dances. In their second year of existence, their annual contributions increased sufficiently to cover seventy-five percent of the cost of the tuberculosis program. Some funds were dedicated to sending poor, consumptive children to a summer camp in the countryside.

The community recognized that the Jewish Anti-Tuberculosis Association's services paralleled those of contemporary trained social workers. In 1912 some hospitals, including MGH, Boston City Hospital, Peter Bent Brigham, Carney Hospital, Boston Psychopathic and Infants and Children's, maintained social service departments staffed exclusively by women. Without the advanced graduate degrees and clinical psychotherapy training required today, social workers of the early 1900s visited clients at home to provide emotional and social support. They educated immigrant and underprivileged mothers about child care, nutrition and home management. However, the field of social work was still new; nurses and members of the women's auxiliaries—such as the Mt. Sinai Women's Auxiliary—also provided services to the indigent including referral to charitable organizations for financial aid and employment assistance.

About the time the Jewish Anti-Tuberculosis Association was formed, the Mt. Sinai Association and the hospital's board—particularly its medical executive committee—began to consider the creation of a social services department. Some physicians and donors resisted the idea, preferring to direct money toward the purchase and upkeep of buildings. Others, including members of the Jewish Anti-Tuberculosis Association, urged Mt. Sinai to create the social work department.

As the three-year discussion continued, some physicians noted that Mt. Sinai remained one of the few hospitals in Boston without a social work department. A board member said, "No hospital has the clientele representing such a large proportion of people whose incomes are of the smallest and whose medical complaints are so great. Yet they are helpless to change their unfortunate conditions." Physical illness most often begets emotional concerns. Fear and anxiety often lead to family tensions and problems. Recent immigrants with language limitations lacked the knowledge or the skills to access aid from community resources. They were truly in need of an advocate and that need was promptly filled by the social work department.

In 1912 a Mt. Sinai social work department was formally established and the Jewish Anti-Tuberculosis Association contributed $1,500 toward its founding. The association made a contribution annually. Miss Ida S. Goldberg, a trained social worker, was hired as the first director of social work. She was to supervise twelve volunteers; some were members of the auxiliary, others were nurses. Some had studied sociology or were knowledgeable about community resources. Miss Goldberg's annual salary was $720, comparable to that of Miss Ida B. Cannon, the first director of social work at MGH. Her department began in 1905. Within the first six months, Miss Goldberg had seen 150 patients, all referred by physicians, and by year's end, 500 people had received social work services.

The Mt. Sinai social work department worked closely with Federated Jewish Charities and other nonprofit agencies to address the Jewish community's social, financial and educational needs. If a patient was not eligible for admission to Mt. Sinai Hospital—either because no bed was available or because the patient required care the hospital could not provide—the social worker enabled the family to make alternative arrangements. When a wage earner was ill and the family was without income, the hospital provided care at low or no cost.

Social workers helped the patient's family members access vocational training and employment. They made arrangements for continued care when patients were discharged from the hospital. Social service workers often served as liaisons between parents and their children's schoolteachers. Such a service helped alleviate family tensions. If language and/or emotional factors involved a misunderstanding between the school, parents and children, there could be significant repercussions. These social workers shared a finely honed sense of social justice, compassion and philanthropy and demonstrated their determination to provide emotional and practical support to those less fortunate.

Ironically, in the face of the Jewish community's extraordinary effort to alleviate the misery of tuberculosis, Jews in Boston had a relative immunity to the disease in comparison to other ethnic groups. Nevertheless, many poor Jews did succumb to the disease within the crowded tenements of the West End. The overall age of tuberculosis fatalities in Boston was between fifteen and forty-five years of age—the same cohort that subsequently died in the influenza pandemic in 1916.

In 1907 Dr. Cabot was concerned about the inadequate treatment of the consumptive Jewish population. He wrote to the physicians at Mt. Sinai, "The need for more and better care for Jewish consumptives of Boston is a pressing one. Especially the early curable cases and the bedridden advanced cases that are not properly cared for. We are treating a great many Jewish consumptives here [at MGH] but due to the language barrier, we are not treating them as thoroughly or efficiently as we should. There is a great need for a Jewish physician with the means—one thousand dollars a year—to carry on a clinic for Jewish consumptives. A nurse has to visit and supervise patients in the details of home treatment, since most of them can't leave home and she is the chief expense.

"I have heard that Drs. Linenthal and Mendelsohn of the Mt. Sinai hospital are ready to provide their services in managing such a Tuberculosis Clinic for Jewish people. I have known both these men intimately and watched their work. They are both medically competent and by reason of their sociological interest, they would be able manage such a clinic. I sincerely hope it will be started."

Within one month, Dr. Cabot received a response to his recommendation. Aided by the women volunteers, the Mt. Sinai dispensaries' clinics began a program. Since physicians most often saw patients in a clinic, nurses undertook the important home visits to tubercular patients. Not only did they tend to be nurturing by nature, but they also had been trained in hands-on, bedside care. They were able to be more flexible than doctors and were usually less intimidating to patients. They identified with the women at home, who were the primary caretakers responsible for household chores and child-rearing as well as the care of tuberculosis patients.

In the Mt. Sinai program, a nurse visited each patient at home to supervise the activities of his or her daily life and offer support to the family. She evaluated the patient's home conditions, made certain the prescribed treatment was followed, educated the family about proper hygiene and, when necessary, referred the patient or a family member to an appropriate nonprofit agency for additional help. The program was successful, showing recovery results comparable to the best sanatoria.

Despite its relocation to Staniford Street and its expansion, the Mt. Sinai Association had yet to achieve its original vision of an inpatient and outpatient general hospital to serve the Jewish immigrant community and others in need. In 1911 a group of twenty-eight doctors, businessmen and religious leaders, formally organized as the Beth Israel Association, met to explore the possibility of a full-service Jewish hospital providing inpatient and outpatient care. Five years later, the Jewish community abandoned

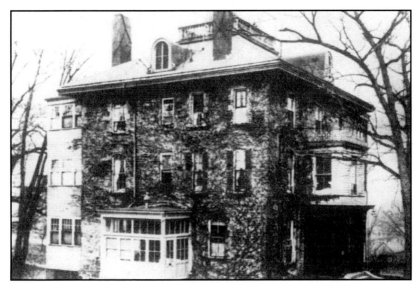

Dennison Estate converted to first Mt. Sinai inpatient hospital.

the Mt. Sinai dispensaries, purchased the Dennison estate at 45 Townsend Street, Roxbury, and transformed it into the Mt. Sinai hospital.

One of the most active organizers and fundraisers of the Beth Israel Association was Mr. Hyman Danzig, a Hebrew scholar and a successful—though not wealthy—businessman. He sold his business and used the proceeds to create a hospital fund. He became the first president of the Beth Israel Association and dedicated his time and money to the hospital's creation. Mr. Danzig died in his late forties, just one year after the association's dream was fulfilled.

Mt. Sinai hospital was the first inpatient, Jewish hospital in Massachusetts. It opened in 1916. The association—which included many members of the group that had launched the Mt. Sinai dispensaries—took the bold step of purchasing the land and buildings of the Dennison estate. It was located in a pleasant residential neighborhood that was easily accessible to Boston and the suburbs via the elevated rail transit system. The association purchased a large, four-story house, a brick-and-stone stable and 150,000 square feet of land for $16,000. The association paid $8,000 upfront and mortgaged the balance.

After its renovation, the hospital included a kosher kitchen in the basement, a modern operating room on the third floor, an elevator, a large, outside porch and forty-two patient beds, later expanded to forty-seven. The stable was gutted and reconstructed into a school of nursing. The Massachusetts Board of Charity granted the Beth Israel Association a charter, which listed 231 members.

Not surprisingly, the cost of renovation exceeded the $40,000 budget. Mr. Meyer Dana, a charter member, provided his personal warranty to guarantee payment. Funds came from private donors, not hospital fees. Since the hospital was a charitable institution, most patients received their care for free. The few private rooms cost $28 a week and patients in wards, who had private funds, paid $21 a week.

On February 4, 1917 the first patient, Mrs. Fannie Levine of the West End, was admitted to the new hospital. Just a few months earlier, the Boston Fire Department had condemned the first Mt. Sinai dispensary building on Chambers Street.

Several months before the official opening, Beth Israel Hospital had enjoyed a weeklong dedication celebration. The festivities included a parade led by a military band and featuring a float bearing a hospital bed, a patient, a doctor and a nurse. Mayor James Michael Curley addressed the thousands who attended the parade. To encourage and support the endeavor, he contributed $100. Whether the populace came for the festivities or to see and hear "The Rascal King"—one of Mayor Curley's nicknames—is not known.

As one of the most colorful and perhaps corrupt politicians in Boston's history, Mayor Curley was born in 1874 to an Irish washer-woman. He dominated Boston politics for several decades. In 1903, shortly after his election as alderman, he was incarcerated in the Charles Street jail for taking a civil service examination for a friend. Some referred to him as the "Lovable Scoundrel" and others as "Hizzoner" ("His Honor"). Whatever he was called, Mayor Curley was dearly beloved by his large, Irish constituency.

In 1947 (his term as mayor began in 1945) he served several months in federal prison for mail fraud. This jail term in no way interfered with his running the city since his cronies were in daily attendance to do his bidding. President Harry Truman issued a presidential commutation of the conviction and later a presidential pardon.

Mayor Curley was elected mayor of Boston five times and served one term in the Massachusetts House of Representatives, two terms in the U.S. Congress and one term as governor of Massachusetts. He lived for politics. "Though he was an exploiter of his own people's poverty, he grossly enriched himself at the public's expense. He lived far beyond the means of an honest public servant." In the words of his biographer Jack Beatty, "Financial self-aggrandizement was not what Curley was about. He practiced *shamrock politics* with his Irish-Catholic supporters cheering him while his WASP opponents *sputtered with rage* for half a century."

Mayor Curley was not an obviously corrupt rogue. Rather, he was an arrogant politician who was dedicated to providing for his impoverished, Irish constituency while lining his own pockets. He acquired a twenty-one-room mansion with gold-plated bathroom fixtures on Jamaica Pond. This was paid for by kickbacks from contractors. On the other hand, he was instrumental in building new schools for children of working-class Bostonians, tearing down slum dwellings, providing bail money for his cronies, paying funeral expenses for the poor and arranging temporary shelters for those made homeless by fire or eviction. He emphasized work instead of welfare and encouraged advocacy programs, particularly for the Irish. Upon his death in 1959, almost a million mourners filed past his casket in the State House.

During the first quarter of the twentieth century, Boston's

immigrants settled in and became more familiar with the English language. Discrimination somewhat lessened and their access to health care improved. The immigrants were disproportionately affected by two connected perils: poverty and disease. Contagion proliferated. Their need for medical care was exacerbated by the war and the public health crisis. World War I brought to Boston the nation's fears along with large-scale efforts to support the troops. By the war's end, families were overwhelmed by the massive number of fatalities. Soldiers returned with debilitating injuries. When the influenza pandemic arrived with the returning soldiers, both the Beth Israel and Deaconess hospitals responded to the public health challenge.

In the winter of 1918, the troops were returning home from the war. Many soldiers were afflicted with a mysterious disease that first appeared at Fort Funston Army Base in Haskell County, Kansas. Huge tents were erected on the base and were so enormously overcrowded that the victims lay on the floor. There were no heaters or warm clothing to protect them against the bitter-cold weather. Within three weeks of the first case, 1,100 soldiers were sick enough to be admitted to the base hospitals and thousands more needed treatment; 237 men developed pneumonia and thirty-eight died.

Boston was the first U.S. city called upon to cope with the influenza pandemic. By the end of August 1918, the resources of the medical professionals and pharmacies at Chelsea Naval Base in Boston were overwhelmed by sick men coming into the wards. Dr. John Keegan, assigned to the base, noted the bluish complexion and purple blisters of his patients. Their violent

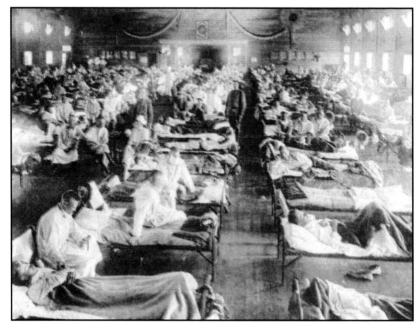

Influenza pandemic. Patients live on cots.

coughing compromised their ability to take in oxygen. Within two weeks of the first appearance of the illness, 2,000 officers and enlisted men of the naval district contracted the illness. On examination of the dead, medical professionals found lungs soaked with bloody, foamy fluid, which remained a mysterious killer.

The signing of the armistice returned additional troops home, many of whom were afflicted with influenza. Along with hundreds of seriously injured veterans, the ailing men crowded into the city's hospitals, including the new Mt. Sinai inpatient hospital on Townsend Street. Admission of 250 influenza patients forced Beth Israel to curtail surgeries in order to have staff and available beds for the influx of patients. Similarly to other hospitals, the Townsend Street hospital reported twenty-five percent mortality among influenza patients. (For a more detailed account see chapter three.)

Almost immediately following the influenza pandemic, Boston suffered a manmade disaster. No one remembers and few may believe that on January 15, 1919, a flood of molasses took lives and damaged property throughout the neighborhood between Copps Hill, Commercial Street in the North End and Boston Harbor. The area was known as Little Italy.

January 15 was an unusually mild winter day—forty-three degrees Fahrenheit according to the thermometers on the freight sheds of the Boston, Worcester and Eastern Railways. Towering above the freight sheds was an enormous tank, fifty feet tall and ninety feet in diameter, owned by the U.S. Industrial Alcohol Company and bulging with 2.3 million gallons of crude molasses. The tank was massively constructed with great carved-steel sides and strong bottom plates set into a concrete base. The previous day, molasses had been brought north by ship from Puerto Rico to make rum and baked beans—a Boston delicacy.

Laborers were sitting outdoors, enjoying the weather as they lunched near the tanks and talked about the influenza epidemic and the Great War's end. A thunderous roar at 12:30 p.m. heralded a wet, sticky, brown flood that headed toward downtown Boston. The phrase "as slow as molasses in January" is not a truism. The thick wave moved at a rate of about thirty-five miles an hour, stood about fifteen feet high and wiped out everything in its path. The explosion hurled a huge, steel section of the tank

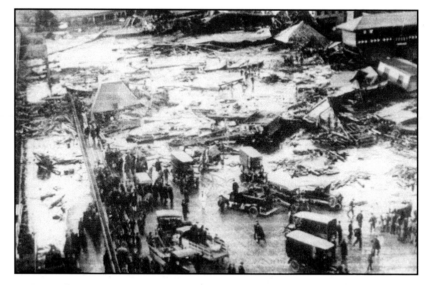

Molasses flood, downtown Boston.

across Commercial Street, knocking out the supports of the elevated transit line. Houses collapsed instantly, killing the inhabitants. A jagged chunk of steel smashed into the freight house where some lunching workers had been sitting. Boston's fireboats, housed near the accident, were rendered useless when their quarters shattered.

The flood rolled over young children coming home for lunch from school. People died when their houses collapsed around them. As it moved through Boston, the wave spread two or three feet deep, covering several downtown blocks. Twenty-one people died—so battered and glazed by the molasses flood that they proved difficult to identify—and 100 people suffered injuries.

Some weeks prior to the explosion, U. S. Industrial Alcohol had received warnings about structural problems with the tank.

The firm's solution was to paint the tank brown, which concealed from view the molasses leaking out. After the flood, victims' families filed 125 lawsuits and more than 3,000 witnesses testified. The court found that the tank's rupture had been caused by a safety factor not addressed by the inspections, and 100 claims were settled out of court. Survivors of the victims were each paid $7,000.

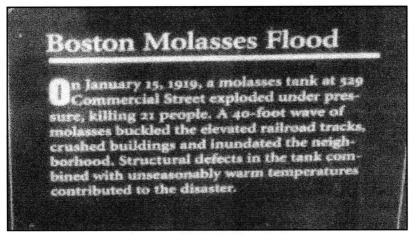

Boston Molasses Flood

On January 15, 1919, a molasses tank at 529 Commercial Street exploded under pressure, killing 21 people. A 40-foot wave of molasses buckled the elevated railroad tracks, crushed buildings and inundated the neighborhood. Structural defects in the tank combined with unseasonably warm temperatures contributed to the disaster.

Plaque commemorating the molasses flood.

Despite the traumas and tragedies of those years, Boston's inhabitants succeeded in improving their lives and establishing institutions that benefited all. For the Jewish community, the influenza pandemic highlighted the fact that Townsend Street could not be Beth Israel's ultimate location. With increasing numbers of patients requiring care and the facility always filled to its forty-five-bed capacity, the first Beth Israel hospital soon outgrew its space.

Most agreed that the Jewish community needed a medical

center that offered both inpatient and outpatient services. Further more members of the Beth Israel Association saw many potential benefits of an association with a top-quality, esteemed research and teaching facility—a train of thought that led quickly to the idea of moving the Beth Israel Hospital to Brookline's Longwood Avenue neighborhood, close to Harvard Medical School.

The Beth Israel board agreed that the hospital had to relocate and build significantly larger quarters. After an intensive and extensive search for suitable property, the medical executive committee and the board of trustees agreed to buy seven and a half acres of land at fifty cents a square foot, paying approximately $163,350 for 326,700 square feet. The land was, and remains, a choice location at 330 Brookline Avenue in Boston. One hundred dollars in 1906 is the equivalent of $1,791 in 2005. The Beth Israel board anticipated a mortgage of $60,000. A fund drive by the women of the auxiliary raised $35,000 for the cost of the land and landscaping—nearly six times the $6,000 they had pledged to raise.

In the spring of 1928 construction was on schedule, but a basic component of a functioning hospital had yet to be addressed: Linens, critically essential to the hospital, had to be in place before the doors opened. Mr. Sidney Bergman, a businessman with considerable experience, was the hospital's purchasing agent. Accustomed to dealing with multiple vendors, he set out to find high quality and a low cost while maintaining the goodwill of vendors. When the hospital solicited competitive bids, the goodwill Mr. Bergman had engendered led vendors to sell their products to the hospital at factory prices. To encourage large discounts, he emphasized the hospital's charitable status.

The Women's Auxiliary, now numbering nearly 10,000, raised money to purchase linens for the entire hospital, from the operating room to the kitchen. In January 1928, the Women's Auxiliary sponsored a linen fundraising concert performed by the Russian Symphonic Choir at Boston's Symphony Hall. Many women chose to become lifetime members, for which they paid additional money and saw their names engraved on bronze plaques that still line the corridors of the Beth Israel building.

Initially, the Women's Auxiliary contributed $8,000 to the linen fund. After that they raised money annually with a dinner dance or other social event. Mrs. Celia Grosberg chaired the linen fund. Her husband, Oscar, was a founder of the hospital. In 1927 Mrs. Gussie Wyner, treasurer of the fund, and Mr. Bergman went to New York City to select fabric at B. Altman, an elegant, Fifth Avenue department store. This first order, for seventy-three percent of the required linens, involved 1,300 yards of fabric at a cost of $6,899.66. The fabrics were of the highest quality and included unbleached and bleached cotton flannel, gauze for dressings, bureau covers, sleeping garments and bathrobes. The fabric would also be used to make sheets, pillowcases, bath towels, face towels, mattress protectors and 300 belly binders for the abdomens of post-childbirth women. The linens were needed by mid-May for the hospital to open on August 1, 1928.

Specific instructions were given for the manufacture of each item. Each sheet required two-inch hems. Some towels required blue bands and others red bands woven at the top and bottom, to distinguish meat from dairy in a kosher kitchen. Lady Pepperell, a well-known name in fabrics, made the sheets and pillowcases.

The hospital agreed to the attachment of a label on each sheet and pillowcase indicating its manufacture by Lady Pepperell for the Beth Israel Hospital. Additionally, 1,300 yards of fabric were ordered at a cost of $4,062.75. Twenty-two percent ($1,481.75) of the order was for 8,000 yards of ten different fabrics. These items were to be sewn, by hand and machine, by volunteer women at the hospital.

Timely—and within budget—delivery of Beth Israel's linens depended on the volunteers who were to stitch many of the items. The hospital budgeted $1,001 to buy a cutting machine, a power sewing and buttonhole machine, as well as stitching and marking machines. A large cutting table was built in the hospital's workshop and 150 Women's Auxiliary volunteers began their first five-day work week as the sewing group on May 14, 1927. A captain was assigned each morning and afternoon, supervised by a matron. Some volunteers cut fabric, others assembled the parts, and many bent over the sewing machines to finish the items. At the end of the first week, 1,452 kitchen towels had been completed. For three months, at the height of the summer season and regardless of the heat, these ladies gripped their scissors and bent over their sewing machines to complete their task on time.

Most of the physicians, business leaders and public figures who had launched the Mt. Sinai dispensaries and later the Beth Israel Hospital were men and women who also deserve credit for their roles in creating a Jewish hospital. Beginning with the Jewish Anti-Tuberculosis Association and continuing through the critical fundraising work of the auxiliaries, women worked without pay on behalf of the hospital's mission. They generously gave their time to raise money and advocate for public health and the hospital brought health care and health education to the under-served. Many of these women took on hospital-related work in addition to their personal responsibilities of household management, child rearing and caring for their families.

Among the women who made significant contributions, Jennie Loitman Barron stands out. Judge Barron was born in 1891 in Boston's West End, the third of four daughters born to Russian immigrants Fannie and Morris Loitman. Jennie's mother was said to be a remarkable woman who spoke five languages and helped new immigrants as an interpreter. Her father was a charter member of the Hebrew Progressive Lodge, an organization with leftist leanings. He took great pleasure in bringing Jennie, the apple of his eye, to his lodge meetings, where she recited poetry for his friends.

In the first quarter of the twentieth century, few women expected an education beyond high school other than for nursing, bookkeeping or teaching. Jennie had much grander goals. Completing requirements for a bachelor's degree from Boston University in 1911, she went on to earn two advanced law degrees by 1914. She financed her education by teaching Americanization classes and working in the Women's Educational and Industrial Union's department of law.

The Women's Educational and Industrial Union and Jennie Barron were a good match. In 1877, Dr. Harriet Clisby, one of the first women physicians to practice in the U.S., had established the union to address the social problems facing women. Her mission was to "increase fellowship among women and promote the best practical methods for securing their educational, industrial, and social advancement." The union opened a store in Boston that enabled women to support themselves by selling homemade crafts

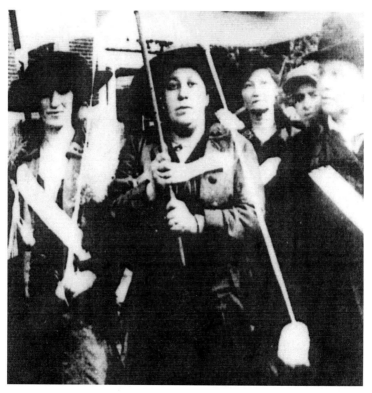

Suffragettes.

such as crocheted items, doilies for chair backs and knitted goods. In addition, the union provided free medical treatment, investigated working conditions in shops and industrial facilities and offered free courses on topics ranging from the fundamentals of domestic service to interior decorating and probation work for the courts. The union taught women skills to work in shoe and boot factories, to teach school and to make dresses that sold in retail stores.

The union dispensed legal advice through its protective committee, in which Jennie participated. At Boston University's

League for Equal Suffrage, she was an active and vocal suffragette. She marched, lobbied and lectured in support of equal rights for women, including the right to become a notary public, which she won in 1918. She worked to affect uniform marriage and divorce laws—previously, women had been denied equal rights with men in divorce settlements—and helped obtain the right of women to sit on juries. She could never abide discrimination.

Jennie married Samuel Barron, Jr., a distant relative, in 1918. He graduated from Harvard Law School and they opened a joint legal practice, Barron and Barron. The couple had three daughters: Erma, Deborah and Joy. Jennie Loitman Barron was the first woman appointed as an associate of the Boston Municipal Court and was the first woman to serve as a full-time judge in that court, where she served for twenty years. In 1934 she was appointed as a judge of the Massachusetts Superior Court—the first woman in that role in her lifetime, she gathered many additional firsts: first president of the Beth Israel Women's Auxiliary, first woman on the Beth Israel board of trustees and first woman on the board of Brandeis University. The National Board of Hadassah and the National Conference of Christians and Jews also benefited from Jennie's membership.

While a member of the Beth Israel board of trustees, Judge Barron objected to a plan that would impose a mandatory limit on the number of women who could serve on the board. Owing to her persuasiveness and persistence, no limit was ever set. She felt the same way about juries and thought that mixed-gender juries would bring a deeper understanding and broader general experience than could be expected from an all-male jury. However, she downplayed the idea of a unique female perspective and instead emphasized women's professional experience and educational accomplishments.

Judge Barron's home and family remained her highest priorities throughout her adult life. Friday night supper at her home always welcomed the Sabbath. She said her greatest achievement was receiving the award of mother of the year. In June 1968, a week after the Barrons' fiftieth wedding anniversary, Samuel Barron died. Judge Barron died a year later of a heart attack.

As the new Beth Israel drew closer to becoming a reality, the choice of its location spoke volumes about the institution's historical mission and its future prominence. Of the eighteen dedicated men who incorporated the Beth Israel charter, eleven were doctors. They recognized the benefits to be gained from close proximity to Children's Hospital, the Peter Bent Brigham, the Deaconess and Boston Lying-In Hospital. The decisive factor in purchasing the Brookline Avenue property was that Harvard Medical School occupied their large campus just around the corner.

Beth Israel's administration hoped that both the hospital and the medical school would find an affiliation advantageous, including a role for Beth Israel training medical students, conducting research, collaborating on educational opportunities, and would enhance both institutions. Dean David Edsall, then Dean of both Harvard Medical School and the Harvard School of Public Health, was enthusiastic about the affiliation and established an arrangement whereby Beth Israel physicians would hold joint appointments at the medical school. The affiliation was formalized on August 1, 1928.

In 1958, on the thirtieth anniversary of the affiliation, Dean George Packer Barry of the Harvard Faculty of Medicine spoke at the gathering. "Beth Israel became a new hospital not because it moved into new buildings but because it was determined to become a different kind of institution—one devoted to medical education and research based on the conviction that only such orientation could provide the best medical care." He went on to say, "Partnerships flourish when they have the same goals and ideals," and added, "Kindliness, sympathy, and compassionate understanding are vital ingredients in the best kind of patient care, enhancing rather than diminishing its scientific excellence." Dean Barry concluded, "The Beth Israel hospital has indeed been blessed with community leadership and with the service of physicians who have recognized this guiding principle from the beginning."

For a quarter of a century, Beth Israel Hospital was the only Jewish-sponsored hospital in the U.S. to attain the full rank of university teaching hospital. Highly respected physicians were deeply invested in the establishment and success of Beth Israel and all shared a common goal: the best possible delivery of health care.

Dr. Charles Francis Willinsky, a prominent physician in the field of public health, had personal and professional relationships with charitable Jewish organizations. Among physicians, he was an icon. Traveling extensively throughout the United States and Israel, he presented papers to medical societies. He was impressed with Beth Israel's concerns about the quality of public health and the prevention of disease, which he had observed in Israeli hospitals.

Dr. Wilinsky's particular interest was in creating neighborhood health centers and facilitating coordination among the various health and welfare agencies. He founded and directed the first neighborhood clinic on Blossom Street in Boston's West End. Previously, he had served as deputy commissioner of Boston's

Health Department and with the support of Mayor Curley, he had been responsible for creating several neighborhood public health clinics during his tenure. Beth Israel's president, Mr. Albert Ginsberg, prevailed upon Dr. Willinsky to accept the position of Beth Israel's first medical director on June 1, 1928.

That same year, just a mile down the road, the Deaconess experienced a physician-versus-administration conflict that gave a preview of the kind of struggles that would beset the entire health care industry seventy years later.

Mr. Richard Lee, Chief Operating Officer emeritus of the Deaconess, initially worked for the Deaconess Association and joined Deaconess Hospital in 1959. During his interview in 2005, Mr. Lee spoke about the strong influence wielded by the Methodist Church over the Deaconess hospital. This became a serious problem. As a member of the association, Lee noticed that several of the association's endeavors were losing money. At the same time, the Deaconess Hospital itself was solvent. Surplus money generated by the hospital was going toward other Methodist institutions that were losing money including a children's camp in Attleboro, Massachusetts, a home for the aged and a nursing home in Concord, Massachusetts.

Dr. Lahey, then chief of surgery of the Deaconess and Dr. Joslin were both distressed that the hospital was contributing, through the association, to other causes at the expense of the Deaconess. The two formidable physicians urged the hospital to sever connections with the association, saying that they didn't want to see the money the hospital earned going toward other institutions. Mr. Lee noted, "When two most senior doctors, who are responsible for probably seventy-five percent of the hospital income, say, 'If you don't end the affiliation, we're going some place else,' you listen."

The hospital withdrew from the association in 1929. The Deaconess then hired a superintendent, Dr. Warren Cook, an ordained Methodist minister with a Doctor of Divinity degree. Despite the fact that Dr. Cook was not a physician, he led all to believe or assume he was. He was a fantastic fundraiser and managed to significantly increase the hospital's endowment. However, in the 1990s, a conflict arose that foreshadowed the hospital's internal struggle. Dr. Cook's businesslike approach to managing the hospital was unacceptable to the medical staff. Doctors felt that their views and those of Dr. Cook were diametrically opposed. They thought he was looking to build an empire, concerned only with his own interests, he was a threat to physicians. Dr. Lahey presented his presidential address to the New England Surgical Association in 1932 and cautioned against the growing authority of superintendents.

One major bone of contention between Dr. Cook and Deaconess physicians was his suggestion to the board of trustees that wards be established at the Deaconess wherein the administration and the doctors worked together to determine and collect their respective fees. As members of the board of trustees, the doctors rebelled when they found out that they did not have complete control of the hospital, as they had thought. Lay trustees and administrators became aware that doctors could also look out for their own self-interests and pay no mind to the hospital's finances.

In the 1930s, Dr. Joslin received a bequest of $250,000 from Mr. George Baker, a wealthy, New York banker, for the construction of a patient care and research building. Dr. Joslin and his staff were internationally recognized; they made major contributions and provided life-saving care to those afflicted with diabetes and improved their quality of life. Another patron donated funds for the Palmer building. Now the Deaconess had three buildings—quite an accomplishment for a hospital that began as a fourteen-bed brownstone.

Chapter Three

To Touch,
Perhaps to Heal

"To cure sometimes, to relieve often, and to comfort always."
—Anonymous

Nineteenth century health care was abysmally poor in America's cities, particularly for immigrants who arrived from Europe and Ireland with just the clothes on their backs. Of necessity, the newcomers lived in cramped, unhealthful housing and survived on meager, nutritionally inadequate diets. Disease spread rapidly. By the turn of the twentieth century even the most indigent immigrants benefited from a steady expansion of hospitals with inpatient, outpatient and community outreach services. As access to health care improved so did the immigrants' health.

The Deaconess Hospital and Beth Israel's precursor, the medical facilities at Mt. Sinai dispensaries, were among Boston's early urban health care providers. From the day each opened its doors, nurses were as integral to patient care as are the struts to the Brooklyn

Bridge. Then, as now, nurses provided the constant, visible, caring presence in a hospital setting that ensured the personal attention that every patient needed. The role of physicians, particularly surgeons, neither required nor allowed for much face-to-face time with patients. A bedside nurse, however, had the opportunity to know each patient as an individual and attend to her or his medical, emotional and even religious or spiritual needs.

Nurses' educations, salaries and responsibilities in the health care setting have changed dramatically over the last century. As the nursing vocation became professionalized and its training programs more academically rigorous, many who trained as bedside nurses progressed into senior faculty positions. Others lead major health care organizations; for example, Jeanette Clough, current president of Mount Auburn Hospital in Cambridge, did some of her nursing rotations at Beth Israel and the Mount Auburn hospitals. She was the president of Waltham Hospital just prior to its closing.

In the 1970s, Joyce C. Clifford became chief of nursing and senior vice president for nursing programs at Beth Israel Hospital—the first nurse to join the senior management team of a Harvard teaching hospital. Although the profession has changed and expanded, the basic role of a nurse remains to touch, perhaps to heal. A nursing career is much more than a job. It is a dedication.

Before the founding of Beth Israel's Townsend Street hospital in Roxbury, the Boston City Hospital recognized the pressing need for hospital care for the underserved Jewish patients whose language and special dietary needs were not addressed in other hospitals. Morris Vogel wrote in *Intervention of the Hospital, Boston 1870-1930,* "Jewish immigrants were fearful of all gentile hospitals, harking back to their European medical experiences." Responding to these fears, two wards were exclusively created for them: one for men and one for women. The wards were primarily staffed by Jewish nurses and physicians.

The catastrophic influenza pandemic arrived in Boston with the influx of injured and ill soldiers returning from World War I. All were desperately in need of medical care. History's most lethal virus, influenza, rapidly proliferated, killing twenty-one million people worldwide in twenty-four weeks. More victims died in one year than during the Black Plague in Europe's Middle Ages.

John M. Barry wrote in his book, *The Great Influenza: The Epic Story of the Deadliest Plague in History,* "Deceased victims were stacked like cord wood." Patients lay on the floors in makeshift hospitals or tents, waiting for victims to die so they could occupy their beds. The molasses flood, a manmade disaster, occurred in 1918. Barely a family was left untouched.

At that time trained nurses and medical personnel of all denominations were scarce. The entire city of Boston had only six registered nurses. The Deaconess was preparing to create its first school of nursing and admitted fifty students to its first class—but no Catholics, Jews or blacks. They admitted only Anglo Saxons. Many students came from small, New England towns. It was not until the late 1940s that the Massachusetts Commission Against Discrimination asked the Deaconess nursing school to remove its "Protestants only" restriction.

In contrast, and in keeping with the Beth Israel Hospital trustees' philosophy, the Beth Israel Nursing School never excluded any student due to race, religion or creed.

Unfortunately, though many young, Jewish women desired careers in nursing, they were unable to gain admission to established nursing schools because of their ethnicity. The schools at the Massachusetts General and Brigham and Women's hospitals rarely accepted Jewish nursing students. Other schools had very small, fixed quotas for admission of Jewish trainees. The charter of the New England Hospital for Women and Children allowed one black person and one Jew to be admitted to the nursing school each year.

The trustees and the Women's Auxiliary of the original Mt. Sinai dispensaries mobilized their resources and purchased the Dennison estate on Townsend Street. The large, brick stable was gutted and reconfigured and became the school of nursing. In the main house, they had forty-two inpatient beds, operating suites, an elevator and a kitchen. No effort was spared to equip the school with the latest, most modern facilities for teaching, including a fully equipped laboratory. The hospital's extensive variety of medical and surgical patients provided opportunities for each nursing student to acquire practical training.

Each hospital had established its own highly respected school of nursing and each considered its nurses the marrow of the hospital's bones. Beth Israel's longtime president, Dr. Mitchell Rabkin, remarked in 2003 that the hospital was, at its core, a nursing institution. Both hospitals were grounded in a religious legacy that informed the education and the role of nurses. In the early years of Boston's Mt. Sinai dispensaries, many of the nurses not only spoke and understood Yiddish but were familiar with kosher diets, Jewish traditions and biblical laws. When recent immigrants received care from a Jewish nurse, they gained a feeling of personal safety and comfort so vital to recovery.

At the same time, Deaconess nurses were charged with a mission both religious and medical. Until 1918, the curriculum of the nineteenth-century Deaconess Order Training School included mandatory, weekly attendance at chapel services and a preponderance of religious courses. Ethics and practical theology were taught along with convalescent cooking. Graduates traditionally dispensed spiritual consolation along with health care.

In those early years, many Jewish mothers disapproved of their daughters' interests in nursing careers. An editorial in *The Jewish Advocate* newspaper in April 1919 said, "Jews are philanthropic and sympathetic as a race, yet they were the last to overcome the old-fashioned prejudice against nursing." Many considered a nursing career akin to entering a convent or becoming a domestic servant. Most parents preferred their daughters to do respectable work in shops, to learn bookkeeping or stenography, or to teach.

A different attitude also took hold in the same community when many working-class, Jewish parents encouraged their teenage daughters "to work for" humanity in the fight against tuberculosis. Young women who joined the Jewish Anti-Tuberculosis Association learned about contagion, hygienic prevention practices and the economic effects of tuberculosis on a family. They visited patients weekly in their homes and helped them and their families resolve problems that arose from the tensions and fears brought on by illness and poverty, which were exacerbated by an inability to speak English. The young women became intermediaries, interceding to improve communication between immigrant families and the schools their children attended. In addition, they approached charitable organizations on behalf of the immigrants and succeeded in obtaining financial help for affected families. Some of these young women later became hospital social workers.

Beryl Chapman, a Beth Israel graduate, entered the school at age seventeen in 1959 and graduated as a registered nurse in 1962, in a class of forty-four registered nurses. An operating room nurse for almost three decades, Beryl said she feels honored to have been named for her grandfather, who died of influenza at age twenty-seven. He had been a tailor who designed and made cossacks for priests. His twenty-three-year-old wife and four-year-old son, Beryl's father, had been sustained by her grandmother's work as a seamstress.

Beverly Singer, now president of the Nursing Alumni Association, matriculated in 1953 and graduated in 1956 as one of thirty new registered nurses. Like Beryl, Beverly worked as a Beth Israel nurse for more than two decades, primarily in the maternity service. By the time they entered the nursing program the hospital had sold the Townsend Street property and moved to its permanent campus to Brookline Avenue, Boston. The first class of ten young women graduated in 1921.

The student nurses resided at the school, enjoying a homelike setting with comfortable, attractively furnished common rooms where students socialized. According to the hospital's annual report for 1918-1919, the school provided a three-year course of education, including training and practice, for women who wanted to be professional nurses. No effort was spared to equip the school with the latest, most modern facilities for teaching. The hospital's extensive variety of medical and surgical cases provided opportunities for each nursing student to acquire practical training.

The board had specifically chosen this location because of its proximity to Harvard Medical School, Children's Hospital and the Deaconess. By the time Beryl and Beverly entered the nursing program, the hospital had several new buildings on Brookline Avenue. As students, Beryl and Beverly lived in Kirstein Hall, a building underwritten by Mr. Louis Kirstein, a philanthropic businessman. An underground tunnel connected Kirstein Hall with other hospital buildings. In winter, a walk through the tunnel to enter the hospital was bitterly cold but the alternative, walking outside, was even worse. Bundling up proved insufficient. To solve this problem without the students having to bear the weight of heavy overcoats, the administration had navy-blue, woolen capes made exclusively for the students.

In that same tunnel, Dr. Paul Zoll and Dr. Howard Frank had their cardiology laboratory, where they created the first cardiac pacemaker. Beryl spoke of having scrubbed in on early implantations. When interviewed, both women talked and laughed about the rules and restrictions imposed on students. Curfews were mandated, as was obedience to the demands of house mothers. Demerits were issued for infractions of rules. Jewelry was forbidden; fingernails were to be cut short and nail polish was taboo. They all had bobbed hair. Nurses were required to stand up when a doctor entered the room. Their attire was blue cotton uniforms with detachable white collars and cuffs. White shoes and stockings were required and the back seams of the stockings had to be perfectly straight. Marriage before graduation was forbidden.

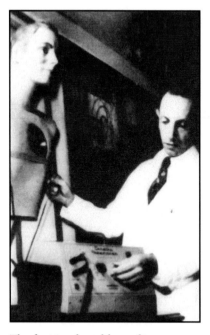

The first implantable cardiac pacemaker.

Not only did the Beth Israel nursing students have expectations of the faculty but the latter had rules and regulations for the students. While the school enforced these rules, it also provided entitlements. Students had two weeks of vacation each year and earned a salary of ten dollars a month. They received free room, board and laundry service. Their daily work shift was 7:00 a.m. to 7:00 p.m. with two hours a day off duty, and they had one afternoon each week starting at noon. When her training was completed and her examinations passed, the student received a diploma that credentialed her as a registered nurse.

Beverly and Beryl's enthusiasm when talking about their student days was rich with stories punctuated by humor and laughter as they described the restrictions placed on them as probies (undergraduates). Two months' probation was required at the start of the nursing program. Beverly spoke of the close relationships forged and maintained with their classmates and referred to the group as "a family." To date, a group of eight to ten graduates remain in close contact. If a member of the group has a problem, illness or other urgent need, a phone call brings at least one of them to the door of the person in need. The group continues to meet for dinner every six weeks. Beryl commented that the alumnae didn't know each other in nursing school other than those who were one year ahead, and were referred to as our "big sisters." She added, "You were the big sister to the class behind. It's a very close family."

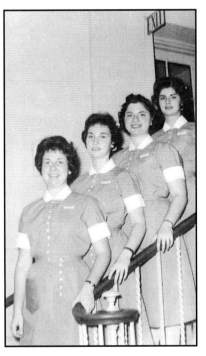

Beth Israel student nurses.

Though there were similarities between the Beth Israel and Deaconess schools of nursing there were also notable differences. Both were established to provide training for nurses for the Boston population at large. Their shared values of compassion, dedication, consideration and respect were the nucleus of the hospital. Each, however, held different religious beliefs and were of disparate cultures. Deaconess nursing trainees and graduates were to provide religious consolation in the homes of critically ill patients while Beth Israel students worked exclusively within the hospital, providing bedside care. Originally, the Deaconess was a private hospital with nursing care provided by nuns or women who served the ministry. The Massachusetts Nurses Association issued a report in 1910 stating that only Deaconess student nurses worked within the hospital, and that they were, in essence, indentured servants. For many graduates the natural career path led not to hospital nursing but rather to home care for private, wealthy patients.

A major difference between the two hospitals was their religious underpinnings. In 1836 a Lutheran pastor, Theodor Fliedler, and his wife, Federika, created a small refuge for discharged prisoners. They then expanded to include an orphanage, a training school and a small hospital. Their vision embraced the Deaconess Order, which focused on training nurses to provide medical care and spiritual ministrations to indigent patients in a hospital setting. Florence Nightingale was one of their students. Some years after its inception the Fleidlers brought their program and mission from Germany to Boston. The school was a major acquisition for the Deaconess Hospital and they shared a religion.

In the early nineteenth century, patients with financial means preferred to be treated in their own homes by doctors who made house calls, and they were cared for by women who had some nursing training. The indigent were hospitalized and the school became a major acquisition for the Deaconess.

In 1915 the curriculum of the Deaconess Order Training School was religiously orthodox and contained a preponderance of religious studies and mandatory weekly attendance at Protestant chapel services. Several of their courses were vaguely related to nursing including religion, ethics, practical theology and convalescent cooking. As a result the school gradually disassociated from the hospital and in 1918, the religious component was dropped and transferred to Boston University School of Religious Education.

In the first decades of the twentieth century the Deaconess

hospital's bedside care was likely to be provided by a student nurse. In contrast to the first days at Mt. Sinai, the Townsend Street hospital and nursing school, Beth Israel students worked side by side with professionally trained nurses.

As the twentieth century progressed the nursing profession became established as one of the very few fields in which women could earn a satisfactory living while providing an essential service. In the 1930s, deeply mired in the Depression, the market for trained nurses diminished, particularly in the area of private-duty nurses who provided at-home care. By 1933, sixty percent of all nurses in the U.S. were unemployed and many of those who retained their jobs were forced to take cuts in salary.

Over time, however, the role of the hospital nurse significantly changed. As physicians performed increasingly complicated surgical procedures, Beth Israel nurses were trained to provide essential services in operating rooms as well as at bedsides. The rapid introduction of medical advances and physicians' time constraints in today's managed care environment contributed to the greater responsibilities assumed by nurses. Today, nurses require higher levels of education and the profession offers a broader menu of specialty career choices than ever before. For example, nurse practitioners—registered nurses with master's degrees—are licensed, under supervision, to perform many medical procedures formerly restricted to doctors. In addition, nurse practitioners not only collaborate with physicians but also have autonomy in admitting patients to the hospital, performing physical exams, ordering tests, prescribing medications and performing some invasive procedures. The number of nurse practitioners in the United States has dramatically increased from 48,237 in 1992 to 115,000 in 2004 and they are in demand in medical centers throughout the country. BIDMC has eighty nurse practitioners who earn between $50,000 and $100,000 per year.

In 1963, in keeping with the need for higher levels of education, the Deaconess School of Nursing affiliated with Northeastern University. Then, as part of the trend in the nursing profession, the Deaconess' diploma students could pursue bachelor's or more advanced degrees. They could enjoy greater income potential and had access to prestigious teaching positions in colleges and universities. Over the next decades, higher education for nurses gradually became the standard. By 1986 the American Nurses Association was advocating for the bachelor's degree as a prerequisite for a registered nurse. At the same time, women had opportunities for many more career options that paid higher wages and were less physically demanding than nursing. The aging of the nursing population, many of whom were over age fifty, presented several concerns such as length of shifts and the physical demands of lifting patients.

Recruiting nurses became increasingly difficult for all the Boston hospitals and the problem of nursing staff shortages persists to this day. In 1974, the nurse's role in inpatient care took an enormous step forward at Beth Israel Hospital. Joyce Clifford, senior vice president of nursing and chief of nursing, established a new "primary nursing" model that empowered nurses not only to provide bedside patient care, but also to work as patient-care managers. Each patient admitted to the hospital was assigned a nurse who had twenty-four-hour accountability for that patient until discharge. The primary nurse developed case-based care management plans and coordinated patients' care among all their hospital caregivers. The primary nurse might expect a call at home or need to return to the hospital if her patient's condition warranted it.

Dr. Clifford's approach revolutionized patient nursing care and her model has been emulated nationally and internationally. Under her guidance, primary nursing at Beth Israel raised standards for continuity of care, which allowed for a genuine connection between patient and nurse and offered nurses greater job satisfaction with the acknowledgement of their critical roles in patient care and recovery. She identified the principles that support primary nursing: effective communication and collaboration among the medical team, appropriate staffing levels, nurse participation in decision making and tangible recognition of nurses' contributions as the hospital's most precious resource.

By the 1980s enrollment in diploma-granting nursing schools had significantly decreased. The Deaconess Hospital trustees authorized their chairman, Mr. Colby Hewitt, to explore a plan for disbanding the school of nursing. Throughout the years, Deaconess nurses had been nationally respected and readily hired. Administrators and employees were emotionally invested in the nursing school's traditions and rightfully proud of its reputation. However, the trustees decided to phase out the school. The last class graduated in 1989.

As government-mandated diagnosis-related groups (DRGs) became a determining factor in the length of inpatient hospital stays, primary nursing at Beth Israel tried to mitigate the effects of shorter patient stays. A discharged patient, if readmitted to Beth Israel, would be assigned the same primary nurse. Though this certainly increased the nurses' duties, they seemed to welcome the added responsibility as an indicator of the hospital's—and the patients'—respect and trust.

In 1994, the year of a nationwide "hospital merger frenzy," Beth Israel was forced to sacrifice some nursing positions. To protect continuity of care in the face of higher admissions volume, shorter stays and a reduced nursing staff, the hospital assigned patients to interdisciplinary care teams. The hospital also restructured some nursing positions so that a nurse could work in both ambulatory and inpatient settings.

A renewed shortage of nurses in 2001 caused backups in emergency rooms. Uninsured patients lacking primary-care physicians utilized the emergency room as if it were their primary-care doctor. Wait times increased along with the risk of medical error because of time pressures, shortages in staff and volume increases.

Joyce Clifford formed the Center for the Advancement of Nursing Practice to promote the professional development of nurses with scholarship in clinical nursing practice. Located at the Beth Israel Deaconess Medical Center, the center promotes scholarly investigation geared toward improving both the practice of clinical nursing and the access to care for minority and other traditionally underserved women. She also established the Institute for Nursing Health Care Leadership, an affiliate of the Carl J. Shapiro Institute for Education and Research at Harvard Medical School and BIDMC. Its purposes are to increase nurses' leadership roles in health care and to promote excellence in nursing policy, practice and education through professional collaborations.

Increasingly, the press informs us of a current nursing shortages that promises to be even more severe, and of longer duration, than in the past. Charles E. Cavagnaro, in a March 2003 *Boston Globe* op-ed article, said that nursing shortages exist because "we never replenished the nursing work force. Colleges closed nursing programs and nursing instructors retired. Now many potential nurses are choosing careers with more traditional hours." And the shorter hospital stays that come with today's managed care environment have increased the need for acute-care nurses outside of hospital rooms, in outpatient clinics and home settings.

In Boston the cost of living—particularly housing costs—is extraordinarily high. Besides dissatisfaction with salaries, other causes of this crisis have been suggested including discouraging working conditions, high patient loads and less-than-optimal staffing ratios on the job. Inadequate staffing on a hospital floor can make an on-duty nurse question his or her own ability to provide top-quality care. As nurses' management responsibilities increase, some nurses may resent spending their on-duty time supervising personnel rather than providing bedside care. Finally, mandatory overtime for hospital nurses has long been a bone of contention— though it was never implemented at BIDMC.

As with other predominately female professions, the public undervalues nurses. Despite the fresh perspective offered by Joyce Clifford's primary nursing model and the current educational requirements for a professional nurse, in many health care settings a traditional approach still defines a nurse's role in relation to a physician's and limits the nurse's scope of care. In some settings, nurses are seen and treated as handmaidens to doctors.

The ongoing shortage has provided working nurses more leverage to seek better labor conditions. In 2001 nurses at St. Vincent's Hospital in Worcester, Massachusetts, went on strike to win limits on overtime. In 2006 Partners and Brigham's Hospital voted to use a strike force, staffing ratio improvements and better compensation. Broad changes in the nature and structure of nursing jobs may be the only way to ensure that Boston's hospitals maintain recruitment and retention of a sufficient amount of qualified nurses. Perhaps the most daunting challenge is to change the negative and gender-disparaging attitudes toward the profession. Greater efforts must be made to recruit young people—especially minority students who have not yet made career decisions.

In 2001 the *Boston Globe* reported that the New England Baptist Hospital began a program, similar to the government ROTC program, that provided students who finished one year at Northeastern University and Roxbury Community College, a near-free ride in return for a commitment to work at the hospital. Some Boston-area hospitals have succeeded in recruitment with signing bonuses of $10,000. However, many nurses seem to prefer more personal time than a financial enticement. To retain these nurses, hospitals must offer shorter work shifts and more flexible scheduling. While one-third of today's nursing workforce is over fifty years old, nurses in their twenties and thirties seem to prefer more autonomy and less bureaucracy in their jobs. Many choose freelancing and work through temporary agencies.

The American Hospital Association recently suggested that to improve recruitment and retention of nurses, hospitals must increase opportunities for employees to be heard by decision makers. Joyce Clifford says that nurses seek a system that allows for continuity of care as well as opportunities to build, and use, their knowledge and skills. Recent indicators suggest that the BIDMC's nursing culture represents an ideal. In 2004, one nurse said, "Beth

Israel Deaconess offered one of the most comprehensive and in-depth orientation programs available. I was interested in evidence-based practice and improvement in patient care outcomes. The fact that I could advance in these areas while I was learning to be a nurse at bedside was the primary reason I wanted to work here. I feel supported by everyone and I really feel I'm a valued member of the staff." Another BIDMC nurse said, "Our nursing leadership team is focused on sculpting career advancement goals for our clinical nurses. To do that, our nurse managers and clinical nurse specialists work collaboratively to foster a practice environment that supports continual learning while delivering high-quality patient care."

Another matter of real concern is the shortage of college-level nursing faculty. Clinical nursing positions offer well-educated nurses roughly twice the first-year salaries of full-time teaching jobs. The Massachusetts Nurses Association (MNA) has reported a statewide faculty vacancy rate of seventeen percent in associate-level registered nursing programs and a six-percent faculty vacancy rate in bachelors' programs. According to Dorothy McCabe, director of nursing and career services with the MNA, qualified students face a three-year wait for admission to an associate's program and the lack of qualified faculty is a major factor in the bottleneck.

A spokesperson for the MNA has said that the problem lies in finding sufficient faculty to teach the students—not in finding students who are interested in pursuing nursing careers. In an effort to alleviate the faculty shortage, the state board of nursing recently eliminated the master's degree as a requirement for the associate's program nurse faculty.

At Beth Israel Hospital in the 1940s and 1950s, it was not

uncommon to see members of an inpatient's family encamped in the main lobby of the hospital. They were usually gypsy families who brought small Bunsen burners and prepared meals for themselves, their hospitalized kin and other waiting families. The family members took shifts at the patient's bedside. Though not medically trained, they could recognize an emergency and knew how to retrieve a nurse. Instinctively, we all recognize the importance of continuity of care and personal attention. Whatever transpires in our health care system, those basic needs remain constant and are largely met by nurses.

In recent years, hospital patients have been more aware of nurse staffing issues that affect their sense of safety and possibly their care, particularly at night. Now families hire private-duty nurses or "sitters" who keep hospitalized patients company and alert nurses to the bedsides in emergencies. As with other aspects of modern health care, our expectations of nurses have never been higher, while the resources that ensure our nursing care seem to have been stretched even farther.

Chapter Four

The Golden Years

*"I don't believe in just ordering people to do things.
You sort of grab an oar and row with them."*
—Harold Geneen

Former Beth Israel employees remember the years 1950 to 1990 as the hospital's "golden years." The staff and administration were young—in their twenties and early thirties—were highly creative and productive, and were truly bonded to the institution and one another. When interviewed in 2003, many still said that those had been the most productive and gratifying years of their careers. Their young, intelligent minds, lacking a rigid model to follow, were free and inspired to enrich the lightly painted canvas of the institution. Physicians, nurses and administrators were peers in age, social standing and professional interests. At work and outside the hospital, they formed a closely knit community replicating an extended family. Many lived in the same neighborhood, their children went to the same schools and they spent time in one another's homes.

All shared similar ethical values and had respect for each member of the Beth Israel family, as well as a commitment to fulfill the community's medical and educational needs. They were cornerstones of the hospital. Like all families, the Beth Israel community included similarities, differences and conflicts. Indeed, factions developed, family arguments ensued and alliances shifted during the golden years. However, if the institution was threatened with attack, the BI family responded as a single entity.

Laura Avakian, emeritus director of human resources, described how the caring values were put into practice. The institution and its staff treated all employees, from the cleaning staff to senior administrators, with respect. While voices might have been raised in disagreement, there was never a personal attack. If a nurse wanted to attend the funeral of a patient she had cared for, colleagues always stepped in to make certain her shift was covered. Staff and employees were encouraged to offer suggestions to benefit the hospital and were not concerned that their ideas would be disregarded. As a result, the hospital implemented many of their innovations.

Ms. Avakian recalled one particular time when the hospital was in dire need of money. An emergency meeting was called for all levels of staff from senior management to department heads, chiefs of service and all other employees. Teams were formed, each with a leader. Each team discussed ways in which the hospital could cut expenses without resorting to layoffs. Their ideas were to be provided within forty-eight hours. More than 1,000 suggestions were offered. Laundry employees offered to consolidate their work shifts from three to two, and they accomplished their work.

This reduction, and the implementation of several other employee proposals, helped cut expenses by $5 million—without layoffs.

Jack Kasten, PhD, professor at the Harvard School of Public Health and former administrator at Beth Israel, recalled, when interviewed, a memorable day in the hospital's history. On July 1, 1966, Dr. Mitchell Rabkin, an endocrinologist at Massachusetts General Hospital, had become president and CEO of the hospital. The same day, Dr. Jacob Fine, chief of surgery, reached the age of mandatory retirement and had to vacate his office. He refused to leave. The long-awaited incoming chief of surgery, Dr. William Silen, had arrived as scheduled and required access to his office. Meanwhile, new hospital staff residents and interns had arrived for orientation and a tour of the hospital. Concurrently, Medicare and Medicaid insurance had gone into effect the very same day. This had been a national windfall for hospitals throughout the country, a major source of income in the form of federal reimbursement for medical care for the elderly and indigent. Adding to the excitement and confusion, Dr. Kasten remembered, the press had called nonstop. He said, "All in all, it was a fun day."

Dr. Kasten related another event illustrative of Beth Israel Hospital's family spirit. At 7:00 a.m. on June 5, 1967, he had arrived at the hospital without having heard the news that the Six Day War in Israel had just begun. He had been called to Dr. Silen's office, where Dr. Rabkin and six Israeli surgical residents had gathered. There was no question that the surgical residents had to return to Israel immediately to serve their country. Jack Kasten asked Dr. Silen if he could arrange for Beth Israel's attending surgeons to cover the Israeli doctors' duties and patients during their absence. Dr.

Silen's response had been, "Of course." With the support of hospital administration, Dr. Kasten had arranged for the continuance of the Israeli doctors' stipends to ensure income for their families who remained in Boston. They had no local relatives and were in need of support. One of the residents had asked Dr. Kasten whether he needed approval to make that decision and he'd said, "I'll put my job on the line." Within three hours the hospital had chartered an airplane for the Israelis' flight home. All paperwork was completed, including powers of attorney, to protect the legal rights of the doctors' families left behind in the U.S. and the residents had flown to Israel.

While many of the Beth Israel attending surgeons had covered for the Israeli residents, Drs. Rabkin, Silen, Kasten, Koufman and others had assumed responsibility for the absent residents' families. Each of these Beth Israel doctors essentially adopted a family for the duration of the war, providing emotional support and forming close friendships. Many of those friendships endured for decades. The Beth Israel families had spoken daily with the residents' families and regularly shared meals together. No family had been left alone. At the war's end, all the Israeli doctors had returned to Beth Israel and completed their training. Then, with their families, they had returned home to practice medicine in Israel. To this day many remain in contact with those who had supported them, and their families, during the 1967 Seven Day War.

Shortly after his appointment as president, Dr. Rabkin designed a plan for community members to join the Beth Israel family. He was well aware that many Boston hospitals actively sought and recruited philanthropic partners for their medical institutions.

While he too was interested in donors, his view was broader and not primarily financial. He invited the support of a generation of Jewish businessmen now in their thirties and forties. While they had been identified with the hospital and had become dependable donors, this cohort had not as yet contributed their own professional expertise and business acumen.

To convert this untapped resource into a valuable asset, Dr. Rabkin formed the Young Executives Group—a reservoir of hospital leaders. His stated goal was "to interest a group of young men in the programs and problems of the hospital and to utilize the skills of members in solving specific problems encountered in running the hospital." As a highly respected, well-educated, honorable and creative member of their own community, Dr. Rabkin easily attracted the interest of twenty-five young, Jewish men. In return for their involvement, the young executives would gain an understanding of the intricacies of managing a multimillion-dollar medical institution with many hundreds of employees. On-site at Beth Israel, they would have an opportunity to study the hospital's operations, challenges and problems as well as share their own practical business acumen.

The group met monthly, October through June, in the late afternoon. They decided that the program required a two-year commitment and aimed to bring in ten to fifteen new members each year to retain the vibrancy of the group and expand its ability to serve the hospital. A self-evaluation in the summer of 1963 convinced the young executives to continue their program. The members attended nine seminars a year at Beth Israel and met regularly with chiefs of service, department heads and hospital administrators. They learned a great deal from staff and from tours of the hospital's laboratories, emergency room and operating suites.

Several young executives contributed their time, knowledge and experience gleaned from their own careers and focused on specific hospital problems. A common complaint from patients was that meals were often delivered lukewarm or cold. This was primarily due to a single food preparation area for distribution of meals. Patients were located in several buildings and on several floors. Mr. Stephen Sonnabend, a senior hotel executive, made a thoughtful on-site study of the food preparation and distribution system. He made specific suggestions and described how they could be implemented. Through his efforts, food service significantly improved as did patient satisfaction. Decreasing costs were a bonus.

Mr. Louis Schwartz, an insurance executive, carefully reviewed the hospital's insurance coverage. He suggested several major changes that resulted in far better coverage and greater protection for the hospital and staff at less cost. In addition his recommendations significantly expanded employee benefits, thereby improving employee satisfaction.

Young executives who completed an initial two-year program graduated to associate status. By 1965 one-third of the original group had served on standing committees of the Beth Israel Hospital Board of Trustees and six former members had joined the board. Recommendations generated by young executives remain to this day an integral part of the hospital's infrastructure: the creation of a year-end appeal, the new insurance structure and the development of the insurance and personnel committees of the board.

This unique training program for community leaders attracted the attention of hospitals throughout the region. In 1965 a blue-ribbon exhibit honored the young executives at the annual New England Hospital Association assembly. Though the group subsequently disbanded for reasons unknown, both the individual participants and the hospital benefited from its existence. Many young executives retained a lifelong connection with the Beth Israel as trustees and donors.

In keeping with the growth, creativity and outreach fostered by Beth Israel Hospital, the hospital annexed a small, private, primary-care medical practice: the Urban Medical Group. Their practice provided medical care for geriatric patients, a segment of the population that had not received treatment as a special group with illnesses and problems unique to their aging. When the Urban Medical Group approached Dr. Rabkin for startup money, he accepted the offer. Beth Israel would subsidize the group and in return, the hospital would become the primary inpatient facility focused on geriatric patients.

The Urban Medical Group aimed to consolidate the medical care of frail, elderly patients in a single health care setting. Patient care and the daily lives of patients' families suffered when elderly patients were treated in a variety of clinics, doctor's offices and unconnected facilities. Care was compromised when patients were seen in multiple, facilities, thereby interrupting continuity of care. The Urban Medical Group instituted home visits for housebound or difficult-to-transport patients—an uncommon practice in the

1970s—to spare elders being moved from one facility to another. Collaborating with Beth Israel, the Urban Medical Group piloted a fifteen-bed unit to provide acute care for the vulnerable elderly (ACOVE). Elderly patients with acute illnesses are at risk for disorientation, anxiety, bed sores and overall further declining health while hospitalized. ACOVE provided specialized care for the hospitalized elderly and later added a transition program for elders in need of post-acute nursing care at home. The success of the joint venture of Urban Medical and Beth Israel was even greater than anticipated, with plans and protocols that significantly improved elder care.

A nursing shortage was alleviated when Dr. Rabkin promoted a preschool day-care program on campus for nurses' and staff's children. The children were in a safe environment and were well cared for by a trained staff. Mothers could visit their children during the day. The program made it possible for women to return to the workforce.

In keeping with his concern for the comfort and well-being of his staff, Dr. Rabkin took issue with the existence of two separate dining rooms—one for physicians and another for employees and staff. The doctors' cafeteria was light, nicely appointed and lightly occupied. The employee cafeteria, though larger, was not as cheerful or well-appointed. It often had a long line of employees waiting to pick up their meals. Finding the arrangement unacceptable, Dr. Rabkin had the walls dividing the two rooms removed, creating one large, pleasant room.

One Saturday morning Dr. Rabkin noticed a gentleman in the cafeteria eating lunch alone. When Dr. Rabkin asked to join him, a conversation ensued. The employee said he'd cleaned offices and corridors at Children's Hospital for twenty-four years and at Beth Israel for twenty-one years. He worked two shifts a day. Visibly proud, he talked of his children, all with educations and some with advanced degrees.

Dr. Rabkin's insistence on respect for each person in the hospital family prompted him to create a patient's bill of rights in 1972—the first such proclamation published in the U.S. that recognized hospitalized patients' inalienable rights to respect, privacy and information about their medical condition. The document acknowledged that patients had the right to leave the hospital even against medical advice and to request financial aid. The document is now incorporated in the general laws of Massachusetts.

1. You have the right to receive medical care that meets the highest standards of BIDMC regardless of your race, religion, national origin, disability or handicap, gender, sexual orientation, age, military service or the source of payment for your care.

2. You have the right to life-saving treatment in an emergency without discrimination due to economic status or source of payment and to treatment that is not delayed by discussion of source of payment.

3. You have the right to be treated respectfully by others and to be addressed by your name without undue familiarity.

4. You have the right to privacy within the capacity of the medical center.

5. You have the right to seek and receive all information necessary for you to understand your medical situation.

6. You have a right to know the identity and role of individuals involved in your care.
7. You have the right to a full explanation of any research study in which you may be asked to participate.
8. You have the right to leave the medical center even if your doctors advise against it, unless you have an infectious disease that may influence the health of others or if you are incapable of maintaining your own safety or the safety of others as defined by law.
9. You have the right to access your medical record.
10. You have the right to inquire and receive information about the possibility of financial aid and free health care. You may request an itemized bill for services you have received. You may ask for an explanation of your bill.
11. You are entitled to know about any financial or business relationships the medical center has with the other institutions to the extent the relationship relates to your care or treatment..
12. You have the right not to be exposed to the smoking of others.
13. You have the right to take part in decisions relating to your health care.
14. You have the right to appropriate assessment and management of pain.
15. You have the right, as a patient who has limited English proficiency, to access to meaningful communication via a qualified interpreter either in person or by phone as deemed appropriate. If you are a deaf or

hard of hearing BIDMC will request a certified interpreter from Massachusetts Commission for the Deaf
and Hard of Hearing.

16. You have the right to receive information about how
you can get assistance with concerns and complaints
about the quality of care or service you receive and to
initiate a formal grievance process with the medical
center or the state regulatory agencies.

Your responsibilities as a BIDMC patient...

1. Provide accurate and complete information regarding your medical history, hospitalizations, and current
health concerns. Report any unexpected changes to
care providers.
2. Follow treatment plans recommended by physicians
and other health care professionals working under the
attending physician's direction. Let providers know
immediately if you do not understand your plan of
care or health instructions you are given.
3. Participate and collaborate in your treatment and in
planning post-hospital care.
4. Be part of the pain management team. If you are receiving pain medication, ask your medical team about
pain management options. Use pain medication as
prescribed and provide feed back if certain methods
are not working well for you.
5. Be considerate and respectful of other patients and

medical center personnel. Do what you can to help control noise and ensure your visitors are considerate as well. Be respectful of medical center property.

6. Follow medical center rules and regulations including those that prohibit offensive, threatening, and/or abusive language or behavior or use of tobacco, alcohol or illicit drugs or substances. Help ensure that your visitors are aware of and follow these rules.

7. Provide the medical center with a copy of any directive or health care proxy you have prepared.

8. Provide accurate and complete information and work with the medical center to ensure that financial obligations related to your care are met. Notify the medical center promptly if there is a hardship so that we may assist you as needed.

Dr. Rabkin provided a weekly newsletter to keep staff and employees abreast of hospital plans and events—from where to get parking permits to the progress of research within the hospital. Each week a note of appreciation from a patient appeared in a "Dear Doctor" letter. The newsletter also noted the death of Beth Israel family members who were well-known to the staff. For example, one such letter read, "It is with profound sorrow we note the death of Mr. Max Feldberg, honorary trustee and good friend of the hospital. It was Mr. Max who pointed out to me years ago that if I didn't pick up scrap paper and other bits of trash off the floor as I would do in my own home, there was no reason why other employees and staff physicians should either. Since then, quite a few of us have picked up quite a bit of trash. I think most of us have casually dropped less trash too, and the hospital is a better place for his insight and action. This is a better place for patients, employees, and staff for his good efforts and we shall miss him deeply."

Representative of the hospital's commitment to its extended family was the response when a Beth Israel trustee had a major heart attack while on vacation in Martinique. The island's hospital lacked a physician and all other basics of a stateside hospital. There were two large, open tents, each accommodating more than twenty patients on metal beds without mattresses. The families provided the patients' food. Linens and sterilization equipment were nowhere in sight. In the next bed, a patient suffered from acute tuberculosis and had a slop pail on the floor to collect his sputum. Medication was certainly unavailable.

Without any functioning phones, the only accessible international line was down a steep mountainous road, in the American consulate. A call placed to Beth Israel was answered by David Dolins, then chief operating officer, who ordered a chartered, medically equipped, propeller-driven plane and a physician who agreed to fly down. At that time, however, doctors were beginning to fear malpractice suits, and the Controlled Risk Insurance Company had yet to exist. On arrival in Martinique, the physician refused to treat or medicate the patient. Five days later the doctor and his wife, along with the patient, were flown to Boston and admitted to Beth Israel, where the patient recovered fully.

That doctor symbolized the fearful climate of the mid-1970s, when malpractice suits were being filed at such a rate, and incurring such great costs, as to drive malpractice premiums through the roof.

Malpractice is defined as a "dereliction from medical professional duty or failure to exercise an accepted degree of medical professional skill or learning, rendering medical services, which result in injury, loss, or damage." The insurance companies' practice was to spread their losses across the U.S., which meant that even hospitals facing few claims, like the Harvard institutions, were penalized for malpractice claims incurred by other hospitals. And the insurance companies forced hospitals to pay current dollars toward potential costs of future liability suits. Full-service insurance companies such as Aetna and John Hancock eliminated malpractice coverage entirely and left Massachusetts or increased premiums to levels so exorbitant as to be unaffordable by physicians or institutions.

In 1974 Harvard teaching hospitals paid twenty times more in insurance premiums than in 1973. In 1975 the Harvard-affiliated hospitals paid nearly $8 million in insurance premiums despite the fact that for the previous five years, their claims had cost insurers only $250,000. That year, Dr. Robert Ebert, Dean of Harvard Medical School and chairman of Harvard Community Health Plan—one of the original HMOs—appointed a committee representing the then eleven Harvard-affiliated hospitals to explore establishing an insurance company with the sole purpose of insuring Harvard-affiliated hospitals. A large insurance brokerage firm, Johnson and Higgins, was engaged to do a formal study and concluded that the group could charter an exclusive malpractice insurance company if it were based offshore.

In 1976 George Putnam, chairman of the Putnam Management Group and treasurer of Harvard, proposed a plan for a chartered insurance company to be located in Bermuda. The company would provide malpractice and general liability insurance programs for the hospitals, management, staff and trustees of the Harvard-affiliated institutions. The Controlled Risk Insurance Company (CRICO) would not only underwrite insurance but also function as a medical and educational organization. Insurance rates would be based on claims made as opposed to occurrence. This permitted a closer match of premiums to claims than the Harvard hospitals had previously experienced.

The CRICO founders created a board of directors that included representatives from each Harvard institution and there were five at-large members. Several hospital presidents represented their own institutions. Other board members were icons of the legal profession and the insurance community. All brought interest in both the growth and development of the company and the protection of the institutions and their staffs.

Though negotiations were in process, the Bermuda government suddenly required that the company deny coverage to physicians. This change would have defeated the company's main purpose. The CRICO group withdrew the proposal and within twenty-four hours decided to move the company to the Cayman Islands in the British West Indies—another offshore base with long-standing, sophisticated banking and financial services. Also, the Cayman Islands had no corporate income tax, which saved CRICO and its insureds a great deal of money. The first board meeting was held in the Grand Cayman Islands a few months later.

The formation of CRICO required integrating eleven powerful institutions led by forceful, knowledgeable men accustomed to pursuing their own personal and institutional agendas. The new company had to meet the needs of eleven separate entities. The legal and financial waters were largely uncharted. Yet, these leaders shared a devout motivation to protect their institutions by securing affordable malpractice and liability insurance.

CRICO represented a remarkable collaboration by the leaders of the Harvard hospitals, yet it earned the criticism of the Commonwealth of Massachusetts. Responding to the same crisis in skyrocketing insurance premiums, the state legislature had just passed a law creating the Joint Underwriting Association to ensure all physicians and hospitals access to malpractice insurance. The state insurance commissioner, James. W. Stone, hoped this would be a solution. Hospitals and physicians were in a "pool" and all were to share the insurance premium burden at rates established by the state. This was expected to be the only medical malpractice coverage available in Massachusetts.

In March 1976 *The Boston Globe* reported comments by Commissioner Stone, who said, "The malpractice insurance company set up on Grand Cayman Island by hospitals and clinics associated with Harvard University violated the spirit of Massachusetts insurance law." The intent of the Joint Underwriting Association had been to prohibit risk selectivity—a situation wherein a private company could "accept the best risks and leave the worst for the underwriting pool." Commissioner Stone warned that CRICO would escalate insurance rates for the medical providers it excluded. He noted that the Cayman location allowed CRICO to avoid much, if not all, state insurance regulation and expressed frustration that he had not "found a way to stop the venture."

Today, CRICO, now known as Risk Management Foundation, has remained unique, formidable and indispensable to the institutions and physicians it serves. Performing beyond expectations, the company has expanded services into medical credentialing programs that are continually oversubscribed and today also provides medical and liability underwriting in Vermont.

Indeed, what was good for Harvard was not good for the rest of the medical community. Massachusetts providers unaffiliated with Harvard had to accept limited insurance choices in a situation parallel to that of the patients stranded by HMOs' selective recruitment of the healthy. When looking at who benefits and who loses when systems change, one must remember that altruism is not a common motivation in business. Paradoxically, the entire health care industry serves a mission in which altruism should play a role: patient care. Unfortunately, as the "golden years" at Beth Israel drew to a close, health care was already being transformed from service into industry. Today, successful health care organizations need to be as self-serving and competitive as those in other industries.

Paul Starr posits, in *The Transformation of American Medicine,* that the advent of Medicare and Medicaid made health care lucrative for providers and highly attractive to investors and entrepreneurs. Hospitals in the U.S. had a long history as proprietary, not-for-profit enterprises. As the 1970s progressed, corporate chains began to feed upon struggling independent hospitals. The acquisition of a few nursing homes launched one of today's largest chains, Humana, Inc. The freestanding, community general hospital governed by its own board and administration gave way to large, multi-hospital corporations. This trend was underway by 1980, when the American Hospital Association reported that 245 multi-hospital systems controlled 301,894 beds.

Dr. Starr predicted, in 1982, that when physicians lost their individual practices and joined a health care corporation, they would also lose their autonomy. Corporate managers would set the parameters for patient treatment as well as physician income. Dr. Starr's predictions came true: Under managed care, doctors' incomes are capped, as are the time and treatment they can offer their patients. Dr. Starr correctly observed, in his Pulitzer-Prize-winning book, that the health care system was "broken." It has yet to be fixed.

By the early 1990s, U.S. health care was widely known as the "medical industrial complex" and its deficiencies in serving the population had become a hot-button issue. The Clinton presidential campaign promised a solution to the health care crisis. The next chapter introduces Bill and Hillary Clinton's health care reform, which may have been propelled by idealism but proceeded without integrity. The failure of the Clintons' effort to solve the crisis makes for a sad, costly, and fascinating story: *the Trojan Horse.*

Chapter Five

Trojan Horse

"When you hear hoof beats, think horses, not zebras."
—Henry Smythe

During the 1980s health care in the U.S. experienced a radical transformation from a decentralized system that provided an essential service to a profitable industry. This shift forced many of the nation's traditional, standalone, nonprofit hospitals to adopt a corporate organizational structure and modify their patient-care delivery to make cost-effectiveness a priority. The hospital, whose administrators lacked a corporate mentality and experience in business tactics, had a most difficult row to hoe.

Historically, most U.S. hospitals had been charitable institutions. They enjoyed nonprofit status, reliable income streams from Medicare and Medicaid and little incentive to hold down costs or pursue profits. Philanthropists concerned about a community or a particular disease or condition acknowledged a hospital's value with donations of time, counsel and significant monetary contributions. By 1990 these hospitals had to cope with a variety of new financial pressures. Emerging medical treatments and state-of-the-art technologies dramatically raised the cost of services. An increasingly litigious public necessitated that hospitals maintain insurance and a legal staff to protect their physicians from malpractice suits.

Meanwhile, hospitals' income streams dwindled as the federal government restricted Medicare and Medicaid reimbursements to keep the programs solvent. Private insurers strictly limited their reimbursement payments for patient care.

The struggles of independent hospitals presented an opportunity for the largest of the health care entrepreneurs to compete for patients and seek relationships with pharmaceutical companies with which they could negotiate prices. The population was approaching 250 million people, each seeking access to an ever-expanding menu of preventions, prescriptions and procedures. It was an irresistible market for the aggressive, large-scale, heavily endowed corporate entities who were not just cost-effective but also profitable. In a 1980s trend that recalled the surge of the banking industry's mergers and acquisitions, health care became a playground for corporate enterprises and the hospitals were now subject to the principles of free-market capitalism.

The traditional hospitals, driven by mission rather than bottom-line objectives, had to reposition themselves to survive in this dramatically altered marketplace, as was the case in the banking industry, where many smaller community banks disappeared or were forced to abandon their unique identities and merge with larger institutions. Likewise, in many health care

markets, businessmen and some hospital administrations con-
trived to assimilate weaker, competing institutions—or drive them
into bankruptcy.

One might say that large health care corporations saved some
smaller community hospitals. Business-minded management instituted cost controls and productivity measures. They negotiated
advantageous terms with insurance payers, private medical practices, equipment suppliers and pharmaceutical companies based
on large slices of market share and economies of scale. While cutting expenses and building profits, corporate hospital management
also assured the public of a continued commitment to high-quality
patient care. However, new problems surfaced: The disappearance
of many small, local hospitals and the reorganization of remaining
institutions into managed care networks reduced health care access
for many people. Within these networks, cost-control restrictions
limited patients' choices, time allotted with doctors and the range
of allowable medical services.

Overall, did the hospitals' new profit-focused approach compromise the quality of U.S. health care? Many felt that it did. In the
"old days," prioritizing health care over cost allowed a charitable
hospital to care for indigent patients in its emergency room. Today
that practice can cause a hospital exorbitant monetary losses. The
uninsured and underinsured may no longer rely on a hospital to
provide all available, necessary treatment. Now hospitals strictly
honor insurance payers' restrictions on the treatment a patient
may receive before incurring out-of-pocket expenses.

By the time of Bill Clinton's Democratic nomination in 1991,
many Americans clamored for health care reform. Everyone

realized a change was needed to improve the likelihood of reasonably priced health care reaching society's forty-five million underinsured and uninsured. At a deeper and more self-interested level, many Americans could foresee the possibly of an inevitable collision of economic and political forces, which might endanger their own access to health care. Some were already feeling the pinch.

The government's role in health care had thus far been focused on adjudicating and paying Medicare and Medicaid reimbursements. Did the tightening reimbursement restrictions foreshadow a greater, more intrusive federal involvement in health care decision making? Would the government someday offer itself up as the single and all-controlling payer? Doctors thus far had managed their own practices, largely making their own decisions about the care of their patients. People preferred to be cared for by known and trusted primary care physicians; and yet, the family doctor concept was about to be impinged upon by large, corporate health care management. The health care market's rumblings left many local hospitals still standing. One feared more of them would approach the brink of bankruptcy as HMOs continued to proliferate and major medical centers expanded.

Responsive to the concerns of the electorate, the Clinton platform called for a revamping of the health care system. Upon his election, President Clinton ceremoniously delegated the health care reform effort to First Lady Hillary Rodham Clinton. To reconfigure and restructure the system would be a difficult, complicated and a massive undertaking. Gail Sheehy, in *Hillary's Choice,* compared that task to "attempting to reform a system larger than the entire economy of Italy." The nation, however, did not anticipate a process so riddled with agendas and fraught with power politics. Perhaps the worst offense was the secrecy and isolation of the practitioners whose very profession they sought to reconfigure.

The health care reform plan generated by Hillary Clinton's task force provided neither inclusion of the electorate in open discussion nor the involvement of medical practitioners. The Clintons' effort wasted both time and money and was the major failure of the president's administration.

A review of the history of national health care policy set the stage for the task force and the etiology of our continuing health care delivery problems. Following World War II, an enormous increase in the cost of health care services was covered by third-party insurers. Due to wage and price controls that were in effect, private employers began to pay the full cost of their workers' health insurance in lieu of increasing their wages. A fee-for-service system was instituted whereby the federal government paid doctors customary and usual fees for the elderly and indigent and private insurance companies paid doctors for usual services provided for workers who were insured by companies.

On the surface, this plan looked promising; actually, it was a recipe for inflated costs. While recipients of medical services did not have to pay out of their own pockets, insurers covered those costs by raising employers' premiums. Chains of private hospitals concentrated on the insured patients and to keep premiums stable, focused on competing for a larger market share. Today, third-party payers no longer pay the bills hospitals submit, but instead negotiate prices with insurers. Large physician-owned corporations, many of whom manage networks of several hundred physicians, controlled the practice of medicine in their geographic areas and negotiated contracts directly with HMOs. Medicare and Medicaid retained twenty-five to thirty percent of the funds allocated for health care services in order to cover their administrative expenses.

By the early 1990s, health care had become the largest, most profitable industry in the U.S. For example, managed-care HMOs headed toward 100-percent for-profit status. At this writing, almost seventy percent of the country's 600 HMOs are for-profit, as are eighty-two percent of PPOs (private physicians' organizations). New groups of for-profit enterprises began to emerge. Physician management firms gained control of many medical practices nationwide and regional provider-sponsored, risk-bearing networks competed with the HMOs. Fewer people could afford the care they required and many unemployed, uninsured Americans were left without access.

When Bill Clinton accepted the Democratic nomination, prior to his being sworn in as president, he vowed to "take on health care profiteers" and "make health care affordable for every family." Upon election he formed the President's Task Force on National Health Reform and appointed his wife, Hillary, as its leader. She would select all members of the task force and present a plan within the presidency's first 100 days. What were her qualifications? Was this a gift bestowed upon Mrs. Clinton by her husband at the expense of the country? The task force's mandate was to affect massive change in an industry that affected the entire population and generated billions of dollars in annual income. President Clinton chose one of his advisors, Ira Magaziner—a somewhat questionable character, as you will see later in the story—to be day-to-day operating head. At various points in this story one may see similarities to a John Grisham mystery: intrigue, unsavory characters, shredded paper, slights of hand and events that led to the near-death of the health care system.

Immediately after Hillary Clinton's appointment, she blanketed the task force in secrecy. She withheld the names of her selectees and sequestered the task force at an undisclosed location. Subsequently, *The New York Times* reported that they were in Jackson Hole, Wyoming. She obscured the details of task force discussions.

The shuttered process precluded any opportunity for meaningful public debate as the task force explored the crucial issues. In *Hillary's Choice*, Gail Sheehy wrote that Hillary Clinton grappled with questions such as: When does life start? When does life end? And how do we get rid of regulation and bureaucracy? Hillary Clinton was said to have gathered 500 academics, government employees and consultants to design the nation's new health care plan. In fact, it was subsequently learned that 1,485 were members of the task force. Yet physicians, hospital directors, administrators and the press—who knew the problems most intimately, had long pondered solutions and might well have contributed a great deal of valuable expertise—were excluded.

The lack of transparency in the task force process echoed one of the growing problems contributing to the financial crisis in the health care system: obfuscation of health care costs. Transparency is essential to the operation of free markets; they cannot function when prices are hidden. For example, if consumers are shielded from prices that are paid by a third party, they are at a loss when making decisions since they are not adequately informed. The lack of transparency in pricing continues in medicine today even though many insurance companies now expect individuals to shop responsibly for quality and cost. Most patients, if not all, have no concept of the cost of their hospitalization or medical services. At the time, most hospitals refused to reveal their prices. With the advent of transparency in 2007, many of the large Boston hospitals revealed this information in the press and on blogs. Many suspected that a government-run system would have higher costs and provide lower value than private, market-based health care. Only access to real cost information can settle that question.

The secrecy of the task force's 100-day deadline and national anticipation of a major, radical plan kept the press scurrying for information, searching for leaks and following tidbits that floated in the atmosphere. According to an article written by Trudy Lieberman in the *Columbia Journalism Review*, "The task force resorted to an age old Washington trick—releasing trial balloons to favored journalists." Editorials about managed competition appeared in *The Washington Post*, the *Chicago Tribune* and *The New York Times* as journalists gathered details of the emerging Clinton plan.

Of the consultants invited to Washington to offer plans and suggestions, several were proponents of a single-payer plan modeled on the Canadian national health care insurance system. Dr. David Himmelstein, a Harvard Medical School professor whose health care studies had been published in *The New England Journal of Medicine,* accepted Hillary's invitation to the White House. He believed the U.S. could save as much as $67 billion in administrative costs by cutting out 1,500 private insurers and having a single government insurer in each state—a plan that would cover every uninsured American. He strongly favored and pressed for a single-payer plan. At their meeting, Mrs. Clinton asked him, "How do you defeat this multibillion-dollar industry?" His response was, "With presidential leadership and polls showing that seventy percent of Americans favor a single-payer system." The first lady replied, "Tell me something interesting, David."

In 1993 Hillary Clinton's group released a managed competition plan. *The New York Times* and *The Washington Post* featured articles describing and analyzing Clinton's "secret draft," a report of more than 1,000 pages. Under the Clinton plan, doctors, hospitals and insurers would be forced to form partnerships that would compete to offer the highest-quality health care at the lowest cost. Coverage for most people would come from their employers, financed partially by payroll taxes and delivered via carefully regulated competition among large, nonprofit HMOs such as Kaiser or Blue Cross and the for-profit, prepaid plans that were springing up across the country. By banding into large cooperatives, employers would gain the bargaining power to challenge health care premiums. The government would pay the cost of membership in an HMO, negotiate with health care providers on behalf of consumers, monitor HMO performance and ensure their suitability for people who were not employed. The Clinton plan proposed the creation of new public agencies: health care alliances. The new, competitive health marketplace would be overseen by a national health board.

In essence the Clinton plan would have placed one-seventh of the nation's economy totally under government control to provide universal health care, a form of socialized medicine. Indeed, this may have been what the public wanted; however, we may never know. In the *Journal of American Physicians and Surgeons*, Dr. James Pendleton wrote, "Not exposing the task force plans was a major factor in the public's overwhelming rejection of socialized medicine."

Paul Starr, a member of the task force with a long-standing interest and expertise in health care, wrote, in 1995, in *The American Prospect*, "The collapse of health care reform in the first two years of the Clinton administration will go down as one of the greatest losses of political opportunities in American history." It is a story of compromises that never happened, of deals that were never closed, of Republicans, moderate Democrats and key interest groups that backpedaled from proposals they themselves had earlier cosponsored or endorsed.

Health care reform was one of the most ambitious legislative undertakings in the history of our government. Had it been successful, it could have bettered the lives of millions of Americans. However, trying to legislate reform in a strictly partisan political environment in 1993 was like line dancing in quicksand. Haynes Johnson and David Broder, wrote in *The System* the issues and events that blindsided Bill Clinton: Whitewater, Somalia, gays in the military, Vince Foster's death, Troopergate, Reagan's fiscal legacy and health care reform. They said that Clinton should have gone "faster and smaller, opting for incremental change over comprehensive reform." President Clinton may not have understood the interwoven nature of the American health care system and that to pull one string would unravel other parts of the tapestry.

Americans knew how the Clinton health care reform story ended. What they didn't know was the inside workings of the task force, the names of its 500-plus members and their internal, daily e-mail exchanges. However, more than a decade after the fact, 435 pages of e-mails were viewable on a Web site that has since disappeared—all from the task force's period in the early 1990s. The following are some excerpts from the e-mail correspondence between task force members:

November 11, 1992—Mark Gibson to Atul Gawande,
Re: The Oregon Plan:

> *"If you are trying to placate the Washington, D.C. advocates for persons with disabilities, then you have a difficult task ahead. I think it would be damaging for Governor Clinton to be seen as folding to special interest pressure from inside Washington."*

November, 1992—Ira Magaziner to Bill Clinton and Hillary Rodham Clinton:

> *"Major Health Care. New System Structure Decisions. Is this a federal system or not? How do we form the budget to control the growth in costs?"*

February 12, 1993—Mary Dewane to Caroline Chambers:

> *"Impose a tax on health care benefits of individuals who do not belong to a managed care entity and/or provide incentives to those who do. Expand 1973 HMO Act to require employers to offer managed care plans as an option to their employees beyond federally qualified HMOs."*

February 1993, Donna Shalala to "The First Lady",
Re: Health Reform:

> *"I can just imagine two administration witnesses publicly disagreeing over what happens to a particular family. Currently, the plan seems to force low-income families into a managed care system because it only subsidizes the cost sharing levels we prescribe for those plans. Certainly our record with price and freezes is spotty at best."*

April 2, 1993—Ross H. Arnet III to Guy King, Re: Modeling an immediate short-term freeze of insurance premiums:

> *"The proposed policy is to cap insurance premiums at their current levels. Insurers could not raise premiums and would be precluded from reducing coverage. It is not clear what this means. Does it refer to services covered, or to cost sharing provisions? What about the addition of lives to plans: is exclusion for pre-existing conditions prohibited?*
>
> *"How are the new policies priced? The objectives of the proposal are to reduce health care costs through controls of 'pre-payment time' and to use the private market to create pressure for cost reductions. Effective use review takes time and effort to design and implement and is costly enough to make the return marginal. In any case, it is clear that insurers without use review would not have time to implement a plan immediately."*

April 5, 1993—Carol Rasco to President Clinton:
Carol Rasco suggests that the president announce a time
schedule for unveiling his national health reform plan and
introducing legislation. She suggested he take an "action
forcing event":

> "Recent Press reports have created uncertainty around
> the timing of the Introduction of your national health
> reform plan. This uncertainty is having a major im-
> pact on both Congress and the general public and is
> diminishing chances for enactment of major reforms.
> Therefore, this week you should announce a sched-
> ule for unveiling the plan and introducing legislation.
> This memorandum proposes a time frame for meet-
> ing your original deadline in a consistent fashion. It
> also identifies the separate stages, products and sub-
> dates that meeting this time frame entails. Finally,
> we set forth the factors that you need to consider in
> deciding whether you either proceed with this plan or
> alter it in one or more respects."

May 13, 1993—Bob Kazdin to Secretary Bentsen, "Reform
Policy Options To Limit the Growth in National Health Expenditures Through Increased Consumer Cost Awareness"

> "The basic theory behind Administration's health
> reform initiative is that capitation can control the
> growth in the price and volume of medical services
> by requiring the use of after-tax-dollars to purchase
> supplemental insurance."

May 23, 1993—Ira Magaziner to Working Groups:

"On Monday, June 7, we have scheduled a briefing meeting for the members of the Working Groups. We will update you on the progress of the Health Care Reform Plan and give you an opportunity to ask questions. You should also be aware we are planning on scheduling another meeting of the Working Groups just before the Health Care Plan is formally announced. You may want to consider this when making your travel plans."

May 26, 1993—Jay Rockefeller to Hillary Rodham Clinton, Re: Summary 5/26/93:

"To undermine opponents, they must be shown as perpetrators and beneficiaries of the problem. Exposed as divorced from the interests of average Americans. Exposed as promoting delay to subvert reform. Isolated from each other to prevent increased credibility through combination. Lose Cabal of policy 'Wonks.' Motivations and methods are mysterious and divorced from the experiences of average Americans. This strength has been turned into a liability. Before the official unveiling, the Administration has the upper hand. Opponents must try to attack without a clear target and are vulnerable to being exposed as selfish, short-sighted and callous—divorced from the interests of average Americans."

In another e-mail, later the same day, Mr. Rockefeller wrote:
"There must be a chorus of supporting voices. Deliver message with a fire-hose, not an eyedropper. A tremendous opportunity will have been lost if the following steps are not taken before the plan is unveiled.

"Demonstrate independence by publicly challenging ideologues and characterizing those excluded from the Working Groups as 'Professional Lobbyists.'

"It is easier to pin the tax label on the wage-based premium, but it would be foolish to believe that it is going to make a major difference in the debate. Under a per person approach, a large pool of money will have to be explicitly and specifically allocated to the politically unattractive population of low income Americans.

"Since it will be hard for the public to decipher the arguments about any reform plan there is much to be gained by winning over opinion leaders who will serve as judges of the plan."

May 26, 1993—Jay Rockefeller to Hillary Rodham Clinton, Re: "Health Care Communications":
"Before the plan is unveiled, expose opponents as 'professional lobbyists' with values and interests divorced from average Americans.

"Use slick presentations, slide shows, poll numbers, the whole nine yards, and choose the 'salesmen' for

their sales talent. This is no place for anyone with an arrogant or secretive approach. WJC (President) and HRC (First Lady) media events cannot succeed alone.

"There must be a chorus of supporting voices. Prepare events that highlight policy concepts: Inoculate against main attacks, which are reform -will, cause layoffs (small business), we cannot afford reform, (deficit taxes), reform will ruin what is left of the system (choice/quality). After the official unveiling, opponents could gain the upper hand if they are able to determine which concepts and details the administration becomes absorbed in explaining and defending. Insurance, national health expenditures could be reduced by roughly ten to twenty billion dollars annually."

May 28, 1993—Carolyn Gatz to Lisa Caputo, Jeff Eller and Bob Boorstein, Re: Conclusion of Task Force on Health Reform and Working Group:

"Because the task force on health reform is ending, it is important that the White House signal that its work is valued and meaningful."

May 28, 1993—Ira Magaziner and his staff rough drafted a plan embodying President Clinton's final decisions on alliances, proposed price ceilings on insurance premiums and the extent of Medicare cuts:

"Immediately following your inauguration, you formed an Inter-agency Task Force on Health Care

Reform and announced that within 100 days a comprehensive plan would be prepared. After several months of major effort, the Task Force staff has developed several proposals for you. In light of these considerations, we recommend that you approve a three-part unveiling that assumes a Task Force release by May 10 to 15th, a major speech on May 25, and submission of the legislation immediately following the Memorial Day recess. We also recommend that this week you publicly announce your schedule for proceeding and decide whether you Approve, as amended, or Reject."

August 18, 1993—Donna Shalala to the First Lady:

"Serious further cuts in Medicare are necessary to make health reform work, provided these cuts are captured for reform purpose as opposed to deficit reduction. We can then use savings rather than substantial new revenues to half from the centrist coalition of Democrats, and Republicans necessary to pass health reform. If Medicare cuts can serve the dual purpose of meeting entitlement caps and financing a portion of reform, the liberal Democrats could be mollified somewhat. The lesson of budget reconciliation is that a balanced financing package is essential. As Exhibit 1 shows however, Scenario 1 Medicare cuts would exceed the cost of expanded Medicare benefits by $88 billion; Scenario 2 cuts excess expansion by $62 billion. We believe both

numbers are too high. The danger is that a proposal to use Medicare to finance so large a part of reform will raise a fire storm of immediate protest from our strongest supporters. Supportive physician groups will face enraged members who view further Medicare payment cuts as another broken government promise. Almost two-thirds of all hospitals currently have negative Medicare margins. That is they spend more on Medicare patients than Medicare pays them."

June 7, 1993—Ira Magaziner, Re: Report on Briefing on Status of Health Care Reform:

"Our job is to continue finalizing the documents by mid-June and start a 3-4 week consultation process with Congress and Governors so we can advise the President of their input before final decisions are made. The Charter of the Task Force has expired. That phase of the process is complete and the President is now directing the process and will do so up through its release.

"The Task Force completed its deliberations and debates in May, 1993. Five hundred health care experts, members of the working groups, had met behind closed doors occasionally emitting smoke signals for the media laced with obscure acronyms and buzzwords: HMOs, DRGs, Global Budgets and Managed Competition. Had the Task Force considered and dismissed the option of engaging in public dialogue?

*The secrecy of the Task Force conversations sug-
gests it was much easier, safer, and more expedient
for politicians and policy makers to talk about delivery systems, health product procurement procedures,
and third-party payments in private rather than to
publicly discuss the care to be given a desperately ill
child or whether a kidney patient over the age of fifty,
should be eligible for a transplant."*

By evading public debate about options and issues and lacking
input from the "front lines"—the health care community of medical professionals—the task force lost an opportunity to educate
the populace and a chance to gain meaningful knowledge that
might have guided a workable, comprehensive reform. A rare political opportunity to affect major change was squandered. The most
unfortunate result was the missed opportunity for a far-ranging,
public debate about the deeper issues of health care: our attitudes
toward life and death, the goals of medicine, the meaning of health
and the critical questions of who should live, who should die and
who should decide.

Dr. Willard Galen, a prominent ethicist at the Hastings Institute, wrote an article in October 1993 for *Harper's Magazine*
titled "Faulty Diagnosis: Why Clinton's Health Care Plan Won't
Cure What Ails Us." He wrote, "People wonder why England and
Canada can provide health care comparable to ours for much less
money. They use a single-party payment system: the government
pays everyone's health care costs directly an option, though highly
efficient, that we seem unwilling to consider." He suggested that

one reason why Canada and England can utilize such a system was that "their health care system does not make anywhere near as much use of technology as we do. They seem to be willing to settle for less than we have." Another explanation he suggested was "the funnel effect" employed in England, where health care services are free and widely distributed. "In order to control costs and also save hospital space, voluntary surgery to correct conditions that are not life threatening is limited to a relatively small number of hospital beds. This results in long waiting times and fewer procedures—whereas Americans want things solved now and completely."

Dr. Galen suggested that the Clinton administration's unwillingness to confront these issues was a key stumbling block. The task force plan did not confront the inevitable rationing of health care. The Clinton administration found itself entangled in the same paradox that every health care provider faces in microcosm: reform aimed to democratize health care—to solve the problem of millions of uninsured Americans lacking access to adequate care. Yet, the reform effort also aimed to control the massive portion of our gross national product that health care demands. "If you promise health care to everyone, you are making that promise to each and every person," Dr. Galen noted. "And, there will never be enough health care to fully satisfy every individual's expectations."

The first lady appeared before Congress to respond to detailed inquiries from several Congressional committees. Moved by all the publicity and anxious for reform, the public expressed support for the president's plan. A television analyst said, "The reviews are in and the box office is terrific." Dr. Derek Bok, former president of Harvard, said, "But appearances proved to be deceiving." After a year of committee hearings, reports, negotiations and arguments from every quarter, in September 1994, Senate Leader George Mitchell announced, "Health care legislation was dead, at least for that session of Congress." On the eve of the midterm election, Joe Klein, a journalist, told the *CBS Evening News* audience that the president had led the country "down a blind alley."

As legislators began reviewing and debating the Clinton plan, the legality of the task force's actions came under fire, with allegations of White House cover-ups close behind. In February 1993 the National Legal and Policy Center demanded that the White House hold open meetings relative to the health care task force. White House counsel Bernard Nussbaum refused this request. In response, the National Legal Policy Center and the Association of American Physicians and Surgeons (AAPS) filed a federal Sunshine Act to force the task force to hold open meetings and release its records.

Judge Royce C. Lambeth presided at a hearing in March 1993 at which Ira Magaziner spoke on behalf of the task force and made statements that later led to accusations that he lied under oath. The judge asked the U.S. attorney general, Eric Holder, to open a criminal investigation and a suit was filed: *AAPS v. Hillary Clinton*. Perhaps the most persistent representative of stake holders neglected by the task force called a press conference to present evidence of the Clintons' personal investments in health care companies. The AAPS alleged ongoing conflict of interest and influence-peddling by some task force members who stood to profit from the eventual implementations of the task force plan, and implicated White House staff in misrepresentation of facts.

Long after the legislative death of the Clintons' health care reform effort, Judge Lambeth ordered the government to pay

$286,000 in legal fees, which were paid to the Association of American Physicians and Surgeons, the American Council for Health Care Reform and the National Legal Policy Center, all of which had sought access to the task force's records. The judge noted that Ira Magaziner had misled the court in a sworn statement about the task force makeup and suggested that White House attorneys and others had pressured the Justice Department.

Excerpts from a memorandum issued by Judge Lamberth said, "The whole dishonest explanation was provided to this court in the Magaziner declaration on March 3, 1993 and this court holds that such dishonesty is sanctionable and was not good faith dealing with the court or the plaintiff's counsel. This type of conduct is reprehensible, and the government must be held accountable for it."

His nineteen-page ruling concluded that decisions were made at the "highest levels of government and that the government itself is, and should be, accountable when its officials run amok. It seems as though some government officials never learn that the cover-up can be worse than the underlying misconduct."

Health care reform was one of the most ambitious legislative undertakings in the history of the U.S. government. It might have been impossible for the Clintons to have succeeded in passing a sweeping health care reform package. They sought massive change in an industry that generates billions in annual income. In researching their book, *The System*, Haynes Johnson and David Broder had "unequalized access to the charismatic, volatile, and ego-driven personalities who were driving the health care reform process." They noted, "Thousands of businesses had a stake in the status quo."

We'll never know if a different configuration of the task force might have produced more successful results. A broader discussion might have allowed national consideration of more of the innumerable factors in the escalating cost and shrinking access to medical care. Those who depend on their employers for coverage also depend on job security and employer benevolence. Technological advances such as magnetic resonance imaging (MRI) prolong lives but also increase premiums and patient bills. The fear of malpractice suits may drive doctors to order expensive tests as protection.

After the Clintons' failed reform effort some legislators tried to address some of these issues. Senators Edward Kennedy and Nancy Kassebaum drafted the Health Insurance Portability and Accountability Act (HIPAA) bill, enacted in 1996. The bill allowed those who change jobs to retain their health insurance even with pre-existing conditions. The bill placed the regulation of private health insurance under the federal government and limited the exclusion of people with pre-existing conditions and prohibited insurance companies from refusing to renew coverage.

In an article discussing President Clinton's signing of HIPAA into law, Paul Starr called the occasion "bittersweet" and remarked that many who were former health care reform staffers like himself considered the bill "better than nothing." While HIPAA has its merits, it may raise questions of whether it does more harm than good in terms of cost containment since it does nothing to control costs or increase access to insurance. It may result in higher premiums passed on to employees and it does nothing to discourage employers from shifting staff to part-time or temporary status to avoid offering them health insurance coverage.

In a speech at the University of Pennsylvania in 1998, Harvard

University's past and interim president Derek Bok noted a "dubious distinction" enjoyed by the U.S. that persists today: With the highest health care costs in the world, our nation remains the only democracy with "such a substantial fraction of the population still lacking basic medical insurance." Dr. Bok rued the failure of the Clinton health care reform effort and criticized the task force for operating in secrecy. "It shut out voices that might have helped create a more viable plan. Voices of knowledgeable persons in the administration who feared criticizing the work of the first lady, the voices of critics of a managed competition, and the voices of interest groups who might have exposed the political vulnerabilities of the eventual plan."

Dr. Bok added, "The real reason health care reform has not succeeded is because it is rooted in a misconception of what health care reform should accomplish." The task force proposed to pay for universal coverage by limiting increases in spending and with mandatory caps. Limits on spending also meant limits on service. Among the many reasons for the collapse of the administration's health reform initiative was the failure of that initiative to openly address the issue of rationing. Hillary Clinton firmly believed that speaking about rationing was political suicide. However, critics of the task force have insisted that the attempt to sell the American public a reform plan that would rein in costs and expand coverage for the uninsured without acknowledging the necessity of some form of rationing was dishonest.

In recent years, large providers have initiated programs that reward physicians with bonuses tied to measures of performance. General Electric, for example, began a program in selected cities that rewarded doctors who reached their targets. Digitalizing health care records reduces administrative expense, and the quality of care improves with a portable patient medical history, which diminishes opportunities for human typing errors or misplaced medical records. The General Electric program pays doctors as much as $15,000 a year for using and investing in computers. Another plan, at Kaiser Permanente, pays doctors a fixed salary regardless of how many or how few patients they treat and boasts that salary with bonuses tied to patient care performance. Medicare has piloted some incentive programs. In one program, hospitals serving large numbers of Medicare patients received a two-percent bonus when they met the quality measures for certain conditions.

A modified version of the task force's proposal was still on the table in the form of the Clinton/Kennedy health care bill. On June 27, 1994, Dr. Mitchell Rabkin was invited to meet in the East Room of the White House with President Clinton, Hillary Rodham Clinton, Vice President Al Gore and more than seventy chief executives of teaching hospitals and Deans of medical schools. Later, on the North Lawn, Dr. Rabkin spoke on behalf of medical academic leaders nationwide and his colleagues who supported the Clinton/ Kennedy bill—leaders of America's top teaching hospitals who were concerned with the future of health care in America, its quality, availability, financing and critical role in the health and future of this nation.

Dr. Rabkin noted that he had met, several months earlier in Boston, with President Clinton and Senator Ted Kennedy, who had reaffirmed the critical importance of not only universal health care coverage but also the special functions of teaching and research in academic medical institutions. Clearly, the commitment shown by the president and Senator Kennedy encouraged Dr. Rabkin to hope for a national plan for universal coverage that would also support the institutions responsible for the training of future doctors, nurses and other health care providers as well as research that would help us to understand and fight disease and disability. He also noted that he and the other leaders were pleased to join President and Mrs. Clinton in "standing up to be counted for the health of all America."

Even as Dr. Rabkin stood on the White House lawn, Beth Israel Hospital and its Boston peer institutions were all suffering from rapid fiscal decline. Within months, Dr. Rabkin faced the greatest business challenge of his career when two of Beth Israel's fellow Harvard teaching hospitals, MGH and Brigham, allied as Partners HealthCare. The Clintons' initiative failed to interrupt the downhill slide of the national health care crisis. Dr. Rabkin's hopes and efforts in Boston were destined for disappointment.

Chapter Six

On the Horns
of a Dilemma

"If I am not for myself, who will be for me?"
—Hillel

ilemma implies a choice. Regrettably, when the issue is health care, choices are not only limited but also severely impact the forty-six million elders who are underinsured or uninsured. Some lives are literally at stake, with many more too impoverished to purchase physician-ordered medications. The question, then, is, What is the dilemma? Isn't it in fact a *crisis?*

Indeed, for more than ten years, headlines have alerted us to a crisis in health care. The root cause is money. Those most effected are the vulnerable Americans whose limited access to options continue to shrink and, for many, vanish. Providers, payers and government policy-makers flounder about, each seeking to improve the efficiency of the health care delivery system while preserving its quality and securing its own fiscal stability.

Medical care is a social imperative that fills a basic human need. Thus, the health care industry, as well as pharmaceutical and insurance companies, will always exist in one form or another. However, for today's provider, the most efficacious route to survival is not always clear. For the past quarter of a century, medical practitioners and administrators have faced one dilemma or crisis after another by being compelled to weigh the cost of care against quality of patient care. Individual physicians and medical centers face the same challenge in ensuring their receipt of sufficient compensation for the health care services they provide. Large provider institutions, HMOs and hospitals can sometimes protect their delivery of care by leveraging their size and shrewdly maneuvering through fiscal challenges. However, numerous health care providers, especially the small, local ones on whom so many people depend, are not in that league. Some administrators, such as Dr. Rabkin, are at a real disadvantage despite their efforts to function as both physicians and financiers. Now more than ever, they require highly sophisticated business skills to keep their large hospitals afloat.

The commercialization of health care accelerated in the 1970s, offering new, profit-focused business models to provider organizations. Throughout the nation, in an effort to survive, providers merged, downsized, relocated and took refuge within health care networks established by larger, aggressive, more heavily endowed financial organizations. The new models came cloaked in challenges. Many required seismic shifts in organizational culture, which made them difficult to implement at hospitals like Beth Israel Professional staff members clung to their values of respect, a family-like work atmosphere and uncompromisingly superior health care. Like other leaders, Dr. Rabkin was charged with guiding Beth Israel through an ever-more-complex fiscal maze while protecting and preserving the hospital's staff, quality standards, service mission and relationships with donors. In short, its institutional identity.

A hard-won victory for both Beth Israel and the Deaconess ultimately came in the form of a complete merger. Today, the Beth Israel Deaconess Medical Center (BIDMC) and its parent corporation, Care Group, Inc., are fiscally sound—a state-of-the-art health care organization. Unfortunately, fallout from the 1996 merger continued for nearly a decade, significantly compromising what might be called the "mental health" of the venerable, family-oriented Beth Israel. Many thought the merger damaged the cultural integrity of both Beth Israel and the Deaconess. While few voiced concerns that the institutions' health care quality suffered, none claimed that the merger solved the basic, systemic health care delivery issues that continue to challenge BIDMC and many other hospitals throughout the nation.

Government and insurance companies now determine allowable lengths of patient hospital stays for medical conditions and/or procedures. These limits apply for entire diagnosis-related groups, or patients with the same diagnosis, regardless of individual situations or personalized concerns. When a patient remains hospitalized beyond the mandated time, the hospital must absorb the additional cost of treatment. Like primary-care physicians, hospitals now have an investment—literally—in shorter patient stays. Today we have "drive through" obstetric deliveries: Women give birth in-hospital, remain for forty-eight hours and are discharged. Even if a rapid turnover of beds is not always cost-effective and an abbreviated hospital stay sometimes leads to a re-hospitalization, the length of stay should be medically determined, not insurance-company dictated.

Today's entrepreneurial pharmaceutical companies escalate the cost of medications. Media advertising encourages consumers to ask their physicians to prescribe specific, newly created medications. There is no question that companies must show profits for their shareholders and recoup the exorbitant cost of research, clinical trials and promotion necessary to bring a drug to market. Yet the same drugs are far less costly in Europe and Canada.

In April 2006 the online *Health Sentinel* publicized a report in *The Journal of the American Medical Association (JAMA),* which claimed that U.S. pharmaceutical companies spent between $12 and $18 billion each year on marketing to physicians and medical residents. Those funds—about ninety percent of pharmaceuticals' marketing budgets—paid for approximately sixty million annual visits to physicians by pharmaceutical representatives known as "detail" men and women. JAMA stated that the desire to reciprocate for even low-cost gifts might influence the medications a physician prescribes. Research has shown that relevant drug prescriptions written by physicians increase substantially after a drug company's detail person visits or the physician attends a company-supported symposium. Pharmaceutical companies underwrite all-expense-paid cruises for physicians and their families under the guise of continuing medical education. Some medical practices receive lunch delivered daily courtesy of a friendly biotech or pharmaceutical firm. Today we are well beyond yesteryear's promotional pens and pads. The cost of marketing is incorporated into the consumer's medication.

From the public clamor about the cost savings available to consumers who purchase drugs from Canada, one would never guess that the money spent by Americans represents just a drop in the medication expense bucket. Furthermore, while the out-of-pocket savings make a difference to individuals who participate, the Canadian option unintentionally excludes many Americans. Purchasing prescription drugs from Canada requires some combination of the ability to travel, an e-mail address, a permanent home or postal mail address, the acquisition of a *bona fide* prescription and/or a credit card. State and federal proposals suggest specific firms be selected to provide drugs by mail—policies that may create more confusion and further distance the patient from the pharmacist.

The elderly often have relationships with their local pharmacists, who are knowledgeable in managing their medications and familiar with drug interactions. If an actual person is available to answer questions, errors may be averted. However, the system generally is an automated voice—a wholly unsatisfactory experience for the patient.

From *The New York Times* to the *Cambridge Chronicle,* prescription medication has been front-page news. Pharmaceutical quality control and the substitution of generic drugs for physician-prescribed medication has been of concern. Large, reputable pharmaceutical firms intermittently recall widely used medications such as Celebrex, Vioxx and Bextra. Negative drug reactions and even death may occur from these same products that the firms spend millions of dollars bringing to market. Aggressive media advertising has a wide reach. Television ads encourage consumers to ask their physicians to prescribe newly created medications. The few deaths attributable to problematic medications have exacerbated the problem as millions of dollars flow to attorneys and plaintiffs—another justification for pharmaceutical companies' price increases. This is the news that accompanies your morning coffee.

Many Medicare recipients struggle with even greater hindrances in obtaining needed medications: language barriers among immigrants, memory difficulties among elders and a lack of consumer savvy among the many who are uneducated in negotiating the complex health care system. Local pharmacists traditionally helped newcomers, elders and others find their way through the maze. Now, neighborhood pharmacies are closing, having been undercut by chain stores such as CVS and mail-order companies like Express Scripts. The loss of personal, local pharmacists is important. They have known the elders' medication histories and responded to their phone calls for information about drug interactions, and can confirm whether generic drugs satisfactorily meet the prescribing physicians' goals for the patients' care. Patients' health care is also compromised if their only access to prescription drug information is a phone call to an unresponsive, automated voice or being put on hold and then disconnected.

With money—the operative word and *raison d'être*—fiscally healthy hospitals must allow business to overshadow service as the motivating force behind the institution's operations. Their survival depends on it. In fact, all entities along the health care service chain are focused on the bottom line. Government agencies, single-payers like HMOs, physicians, medical specialists, pharmacists and drug manufacturers look to cut their costs while at the same time increase their profits; some grow larger and richer before our very eyes. The system rewards productivity perhaps more than it rewards health outcomes.

In such a climate, Partners, Inc., the alliance of MGH and Brigham, presented a prototype of the fiscally motivated, super-sized hospital. Once the alliance came out of the shadows, Partners rapidly publicized and demonstrated its power and fiscal strength and developed strategies to increase market share. The alliance created special, exclusive relationships with community providers and ultimately grew to dominate the region's health care industry. Private-practice physicians were courted. Partners' network expanded and MGH/Brigham beds were filled. Because of its size and fiscal stability, Partners could broker profitable deals with pharmaceutical and insurance companies, the government and other providers. Growth led to medical achievements, which helped Partners accrue enormous endowments. Their position and prestige was solidified and unassailable.

In 2005 Massachusetts General Hospital earned a profit of $188 million and Brigham's profit was $74.8 million. Under Massachusetts law, as not-for-profit, charitable organizations, their excess was defined as surplus, not profit. Dr. James J. Mongan, MGH president, told *The Boston Globe,* "Partners' surplus is not used to reduce the cost to the patients/consumers, rather to enhance the hospital."

The MGH/Brigham alliance surely posed a threat to the other

Harvard hospitals that were each facing their own ongoing fiscal problems. Government and insurance-company reimbursements decreased the funds available to underwrite medical students' training. Pharmaceutical companies escalated the costs of medication. The cost of malpractice insurance forced many doctors to leave Massachusetts, exacerbating the problem of physician recruitment and retention that accompanied a long-running shortage of nurses. Even Brigham and Women's Hospital searched for two years for a "star" cardiac surgeon. Luring a choice candidate was made even more difficult by the gap between the salary the hospital could afford to pay and the larger offers made by other institutions.

Despite healthy endowments, efficient operational management and a century-long legacy of community service and innovation, Beth Israel Hospital felt the squeeze. In 1994 the hospital was already fiscally in the red. Harvard Medical School's Dean Tosteson convened a meeting of the Harvard teaching hospitals to address the local manifestation of the national health care crisis. Beth Israel Hospital found itself, like many others, on the horns of a dilemma. Without a magic tourniquet to stem its hemorrhaging money, the hospital's management faced painfully difficult choices: sell to a for-profit company or push harder to increase market share and further trim costs. Dr. Rabkin's senior management team and the board of trustees most dreaded having to lay off staff and feared that the hospitals would face bankruptcy.

The Deaconess Hospital, Beth Israel's neighbor and also a Harvard affiliate, faced equally difficult choices. Also heavily in debt in 1994, the Deaconess' bonds hovered just above the junk bond category. After MGH and Brigham allied, the Deaconess board and management feared they would be faced with absorption into the

Partners system. Casting about for solutions, they began conversations with various potential partnering institutions. The Deaconess presented a desirable partner for Beth Israel. Though smaller than Beth Israel, its health care services were held in esteem. The Deaconess offered an outstanding diabetes research department, was renowned for specialty surgery and had its own venerable history. Furthermore, if the Deaconess were to join another institution, particularly Partners, Beth Israel would find itself relegated to a permanent secondary status in the Harvard constellation. By merging with the Deaconess, Beth Israel would not only survive but would also maintain its prominence in the constellation of Harvard teaching hospitals.

When the dust settled, Beth Israel and Deaconess leadership were determined to fully merge the two hospitals into Beth Israel Deaconess Medical Center (BIDMC) under a new parent company, Care Group, Inc. The merger would preserve each hospital's long-standing institutional mission and allow each to continue providing high-quality care. Together, they hoped to have the clout to stand up to Partners. In February 1996, Care Group announced their creation of a health care provider network with more than 1,200 physicians, 7,500 employees and nearly $1.8 billion in revenue.

Dr. Rabkin and Deaconess CEO Dr. Richard J. Gaitner did not consider replicating the MGH and Brigham and Women's alliance. Instead they made a strong, public statement of a complete, integrated merger. A single chief of service would lead each newly combined department, including nursing, medicine and surgery, and all others. One president/CEO would direct the merged hospitals with a single board of trustees determining the new institution's direction. Dr. Rabkin said that by combining all clinical and administrative functions, the two hospitals would become a "streamlined entity rather than a fatter institution." He also stated that Care Group would not reduce staff in accordance with their long-standing policy of attrition, not layoffs.

Amalgamating two distinctly different institutions was much more easily said than done. The first challenge was to merge the structures and unify the leadership. Without a dispute, the CEO mantle came to rest on the shoulders of Dr. Rabkin, Dr. Gaitner, the director of the Deaconess, Pathways Health Network and four community hospitals owned by the Deaconess. They had no choice but to step into a subordinate role. This top-level configuration fueled the impression that Beth Israel Hospital was taking over the Deaconess. Years later, Deaconess staff members who had lived through the merger process continued to refer to it as the Beth Israel "takeover." Within a year, Dr. Gaitner left not only Care Group but also the New England region, taking a senior position at a Southern hospital. The position of BIDMC CEO changed hands six times before Mr. Paul Levy was appointed to the position in 2002.

The merger created a single board of trustees. Mr. Stephen Kay, Beth Israel board chairman, became chair of the Care Group board and Mr. John Hamill, Pathways' chair, became vice chair. With the integration of the two hospital boards, many long-esteemed Beth Israel Hospital trustees were mandatorily retired and relegated to newly created roles as "overseers." Many of these dedicated, philanthropic trustees had, over many decades, served on committees, provided endowments and underwritten construction of hospital buildings. These elders carried the legacy of their forebearers, who had founded Beth Israel to meet a community need. Immersed in the hospital's history, they identified strongly with its mission.

One forcibly retired Beth Israel board member who had been very active for more than four decades recalled, in 2003, "We were dismissed with a thirty-five cent stamp." Another, Mrs. Francis Friedman, the first woman to serve on the Beth Israel board, said she had been insulted by the letter she'd received informing her of her new status as overseer. She no longer had a vote and was permitted to attend a board meeting only if invited. The disrespect shown these long-term trustees—truly the elders—caused deep sadness. They felt betrayed, offended and surprised by their suddenly diminished status and shamed by their apparent lack of value. Consequently the newly merged institution suffered the loss of several former Beth Israel's goodwill and knowledge, as well as a slowing of philanthropy.

In truth, a merger of the two full boards would have been exceedingly cumbersome with approximately forty decision-making members. However, in a gesture symbolic of a corporate climate in health care, the shrinking of the board was accomplished without forewarning. Beth Israel and Deaconess staff felt the merger's shake-up at every level, from management to housekeeping, and in every clinical department. Tension tainted BIDMC as a work environment from the 1996 merger into the next decade. Yet the painful struggles of the two hospitals as they merged were barely visible to patients, who continued to interface with staff as they always had. Though medical care in both hospitals remained at the highest level despite internal administrative struggles, staff turnover did have an impact on patients who needed and wanted the connection to their primary-care physicians, some of who ultimately left the hospital.

Nevertheless the BIDMC-affiliated physicians continued to

work under extraordinarily challenging conditions, heightening rather than lessening the tensions brought on by the merger. While the value of personal connection in health care is rarely mentioned in the public debate, clear channels of communication and a sense of trust are critical, irreplaceable assets to a therapeutic relationship. Without the benefit of modern psychotherapy, the founders of Beth Israel Hospital had instinctively known the importance of personal care and its connection to healing. They viewed medical care as more than a service for purchase; it was an integral part of community life and responsibility. Nonetheless, patients received caring along with their health care, a value the Beth Israel Deaconess Medical Center espouses to this day.

Caring takes time and today's health care providers are stretched to their capacity. Though not solely the fault of the merger, time is a precious and rare commodity even at BIDMC. Twenty minutes constitutes an office visit and some patients feel fortunate to have even that much access to a doctor. Often the doctor is someone they've never seen before. Many patients triage their own health concerns since there is barely enough time to talk about their chief complaints.

Perhaps the greatest loss for both patient and doctor is the diminished time for face-to-face interaction. If a patient does not feel heard or understood, anxiety becomes an uncomfortable third presence in the room. Neither patient nor doctor can derive satisfaction from a rushed, disconnected interaction. When a cost-versus-care conflict occurs and the insurance company has denied approval of a test or the patient is unable to gain access to a specialist, conflict may ensue between patient and doctor. The relationship becomes not just distant but even adversarial. Then, another presence may enter the room: the ghost of a malpractice claim.

A frayed, fractured or nonexistent patient-physician relationship can foster a malpractice suit. In the 1960s malpractice did not cross the mind of the family doctor even when health outcomes were poor or even tragic. Generally, patients trusted their compassionate, personal physicians to do their very best for them and their families. Without secure patient-doctor relationships, some doctors resort to "defensive medicine" to avoid malpractice suits. A physician may order a battery of expensive tests or procedures in an effort to forestall or avoid a litigious outcome. A patient or family not only has the right but often the support of society and the justice system to seek financial compensation for a less-than-satisfactory medical outcome.

Many Americans today find their treatment plans approved or disapproved by clerical employees of health maintenance organizations or insurers. They were expected to bring health care to greater segments of the population while instituting strict financial management to cut costs. An initial cost-control measure of HMOs was to cherry-pick young, healthy, working patients and their families, for whom chronic diseases such as emphysema and arthritis were rarely a problem. However, as baby boomers reached middle age and needed more expensive medical care, HMOs began to limit hospitalizations, deny tests and reject patient requests to visit specialists. HMOs prefer less-expensive generic medications over more costly though perhaps more effective prescription drugs. They insist that patients only use their doctors in the HMO network regardless of the nature and complexity of a patient's problem, or the HMO denies the claim.

Where state law permits, many doctors must pursue their own

patients for payments not covered by insurance. Adding insult to injury, many physician groups must employ at least one full-time employee to submit insurance forms and negotiate with payers. Pediatric Alliance, a network of thirty-seven pediatricians in the Pittsburgh, Pennsylvania, area, spends at least $250,000 a year on the salaries of eight billing clerks and still requires other staff members to spend time verifying each patient's coverage and collection of copayments. They also pay an outside company to check bills for accuracy before they are mailed. The ongoing battle over who will ultimately pay inflates the price tag on every medical service.

Once considered the answer to an elderly person's prayer, Medicare now determines the tests a patient may have and only sometimes grudgingly approves them. An eighty-year-old woman, having had bilateral lumpectomies for early-stage breast cancer, is told on the phone by a Medicare employee that she would be allowed a reimbursable mammogram every two years and a pap smear every five years. So much for Medicare and Medex Gold insurance, the annual premium of which is $4,000.

It is the doctor's responsibility to keep treatment within mandated limits, weighing cost against value at every step in patient care. By skillfully capping treatment expenses, a doctor can turn his or her practice into a profit center. A seriously or chronically ill patient may present a financial liability for his or her doctor, which the doctor can minimize by prescribing lower-cost medication, ordering shorter-than-optimal hospital stays or foregoing an expensive laboratory test.

In today's health care scenario, insurers are metaphorically the chief executive officers of every physician's practice. Typically not medically trained, they base decisions on code numbers that represent the diagnosis. When cost exceeds mandated limits, a physician may risk denial of reimbursement and may be forced to cover medications out of his or her own income. Doctors receive far less compensation than their billed fees and can wait months for payment. Medicare now determines the tests a patient may have. Medicare and insurance company employees have become gatekeepers for the health care of complete strangers. The ongoing battle over who will pay ultimately inflates the price tags on every medical service.

In 2000, a public television program, PBS' *Frontline*, aired an episode called "Dr. Solomon's Dilemma," which forthrightly portrayed, through the eyes of a well-known Beth Israel primary-care physician, the struggle inherent in delivering high-quality health care. The ethical conflicts, frustrations and day-to-day binds confronting a primary-care physician were portrayed in gripping, forthright dialogue. It also provided a glimpse behind the scenes of BIDMC, then in its fourth year as a merged institution.

Dr. Martin Solomon, a primary-care physician for more than twenty years, represents today's practices at the Brigham and Women's Hospital. Regularly, he had been named one of Boston's top ten primary-care physicians. Based at Beth Israel Hospital in 1999, he treated thirty-five patients each day in mandated twenty-minute visits. In addition, he received hundreds of phone calls daily and worked ten-hour days that began with hospital rounds at 5:00 a.m.

Strictly limited time with patients troubled Dr. Solomon. However, what worried him even more was the pressure to keep his patients from seeking treatment outside their provider groups. If a patient did so, Dr. Solomon explained, as the patient's primary physician, he would have to pay the out-of-network doctor and the designated provider group hospital. In this case, BIDMC had to pay the competing hospital. His personal income was thereby diminished, along with the incomes of his colleagues, since his practice group or "pod" bore these financial burdens. "Quite honestly, every single week this comes up, sometimes every day," Dr. Solomon told *Frontline*. "I hate it. It's the worst thing I'm doing now. I try not to think about it. If I can get through a day without having to do that once, it's a great day."

By featuring Dr. Solomon, *Frontline* described the pod model then gaining popularity among the Harvard teaching hospitals. The hospitals were all expanding their provider networks by purchasing group practices and transforming them into pods. Like other private physician groups, Dr. Solomon's had sold its practice to Care Group—by 1999 a network that included seven hospitals, 3,000 doctors, and 400,000 patients.

"Pods" provided the hospital a steady conduit for patients as well as opportunities to improve continuity of care by relying on affiliated doctors rather than HMOs to provide patients with the care and pay for their hospitalizations. While the arrangement offered benefits to both the doctors and the hospital, a major downside for the doctors was their increased financial risk. As *Frontline*'s voice-over explained, "The more care they give, the more it costs them directly. So the sickest patients become not just people in need but money-losers. The conflict of interest now pits doctors versus insurance companies and patients are caught in the middle."

"Everyone's salary and contract is on the line and the numbers are shown to us on a regular basis. Every month we see how deep in the red we are," Dr. Solomon told *Frontline*. BIDMC provided the pod with detailed reports that identified which patients and, in fact, which physician decisions cost the pod excessively. These reports were essentially bills, as the pod had to reimburse BIDMC for some of its losses. Surely a threat to a doctor's personal income can consciously or unconsciously influence his or her decisions about patient care. A pod physician factors cost into any treatment plan. This is not an accusation but a truism.

When Dr. Solomon was asked about the dilemma presented by a patient wanting to get care outside the pod, he said, "They can only go to the doctor if we allow them to go. That's the catch. If they call their insurance company and say, 'I want to go to a particular physician who happens to be out of my provider group but he's a member of your insurance plan, will I be covered?' The insurance company says, 'If your physician says it's okay, then it's okay with us.'"

One young woman had a rare, complicated malignancy that presented such a dilemma. The patient, on her own, identified a physician in an outside medical group in Boston who had considerable experience treating her particular malignancy. Dr. Solomon told his patient, "Our hospital is paying the other hospital and I'm paying the other physician. That would be coming out of our pocket to pay for this. She had done considerable research and thought this was the place she should go." He added, "I understood that, but also understand that I could not allow her to go there."

The patient asked Dr. Solomon if he was refusing her request to see the other physician "because of money." He said she was right. He told *Frontline*, "If it was just about medical care, I'd let you go wherever you want but this is a contract and I'm not in the business of subsidizing your care. The way the insurance company has structured this, if you go out of the provider group, my colleagues and I subsidize your care at the other institution: You're taking money that's being withheld from us to pay for your care. That's not what we're here for. We're here to take care of you. If we can't give you the care you need, then it's reasonable to go elsewhere." She did.

Dr. Solomon lamented, "In this moral real world, we don't have a choice. We have to provide the care but we can't go on doing that forever for everybody. From the patients' perspective, they may not necessarily be getting the best care."

Under the pod model, the group's physicians are accountable to their employer. At the time of the *Frontline* story, Dr. James Reinersten was the president of BIDMC and his point man was Dr. Kim Saal, a medical efficiency expert charged with controlling costs. His staff generated the detailed reports that informed Dr. Solomon and his colleagues how far in the red they were. Dr. Saal told *Frontline*, "The key to saving money is reining in doctors. I think doctors control eighty percent of health care costs with their pens. Therefore, I think it is critical that the doctor has some responsibility for the cost incurred."

Frontline described Dr. Saal's approach: measuring doctors' spending in order to manage it. Dr. Saal's expense-tracking revealed that Dr. Solomon spent more than the average member of the pod for radiology services—on average, two dollars more per month than his pod colleagues. Dr. Saal said, "His costs over the past year have gone from about ten dollars a month per patient to now over twelve dollars per month per patient." Another report showed Care Group's progress in reducing the length of patient hospital stays. His team was able to determine the cost per "unit" (patient) for office visits, inpatient hospitalizations and inpatient or outpatient surgery.

The financial pressures on Dr. Solomon's pod represented a microcosm and reflected the pressure on large Boston providers including Care Group itself. In 1999 Care Group's losses approached $100 million. The same year, Tufts Health Plan lost $41 million, Partners lost $47 million and Harvard Pilgrim—the state's largest health plan—went into receivership. In the documentary, Dr. Reinersten pointed to a "triple threat which results in losses in Boston": reduced federal payments to providers, reduced rates of payment to providers under managed-care contracts and the rising costs of drugs, medical technology, and other budget items.

Following the story, *Frontline* included a segment of feedback from several of Care Group's senior physicians and administrators including Dr. Reinersten and Dr. Rabkin, who was by then a president emeritus. Overall they felt as though the story had fairly presented Dr. Solomon's dilemma. Dr. Herbert Kressel, BIDMC's chief of radiology, said, "I was amazed at your ability to take such a complex issue and lay it bare."

At the time, Dr. Tom Delbanco was a thirty-five-year member of Beth Israel's staff and BIDMC's chief of general care, medicine and primary care. He said, "If we forget to keep our eye on that ball, which is the doctor-patient relationship, we're going to sink." Later, Dr. Delbanco said, "I thought you [*Frontline*'s producers] were fair to our hospital, which was terrified by what you might have done. You were clear in your exposition of a difficult set of issues. As always there were parts one might have done differently."

Dr. Rabkin said he found the program to be a "clear-eyed"

presentation of the conflict that confronts both doctors and hospitals to do the right thing for patients today and yet remain financially viable enough to be able to do the right things for patients tomorrow. There will have to be some limits, otherwise we'll be back in uncontrolled inflation followed by the same sort of onerous dilemmas that confront us today.

Dr. Reinersten responded, "Somewhat to my surprise, most of the feedback I received has been positive, honest, courageous, informative, and I admire the institution for taking the risk. My personal reaction has been somewhat different. I'm still trying to sort out why I feel this way, but I'm angry about being portrayed as the heavy in this story. My read on it is that you used a popular journalistic device, I'll call it 'Erin Brockovich,' to pitch the powerless good guy against the evil big organization usually personified by a man in a suit. I was not aware, during any part of the interview, that I was being set up to be that man in the suit and I must admit it doesn't feel good. As journalism, it worked well and I congratulate you for that and it got the point across."

He continued, "What's ironic and what feels bad to me is that most of my career has been spent trying to remove the sorts of dilemmas faced by Dr. Solomon and had you asked me, I would have pointed out some very interesting ways to deal with those dilemmas. What's even more ironic is that the system of pods information feedback and doctor-led management of care at Care Group was chosen and designed by the doctors themselves long before I arrived on the scene. I'm going to continue to work to preserve the mission of this great institution. I will be working today with a few less hours of sleep and with some unknown number of my staff, who have gained the impression through this documentary that their CEO does not care about the mission, only about money. Admittedly that's a personal issue. Since I'm the CEO it becomes something of an institutional issue because it diminishes my effectiveness as a leader. Only time will tell whether that diminished effectiveness will be trivial or significant. In the meantime, I'll get over it."

Time did tell. He was fired.

So many complicated issues with so few answers. The two largest, most heavily endowed hospitals serving Boston—Massachusetts General and Brigham and Women's—stealthily found their own routes to survival, followed by Beth Israel, the Deaconess and many others. Yet physicians under the Care Group umbrella and across the nation continue to grapple with cost-versus-care questions every day. The money it costs to provide Americans with health care is passed like a hot potato among various entities. The special interests of insurance, pharmaceutical companies, biotech companies, Medicare and Medicaid persistently attempt to establish policies that may not be in a patient's best interest. Organ transplants proliferate and new diseases evolve and mutate, demanding expensive research and technology. Research generates new, sometimes unaffordable medications that can sustain life longer than ever before imagined. Cost and care teeter up and down on their seesaw with apparently no balance achievable.

Some doctors feel indentured despite advances in medical technology, the advent of previously unimaginable surgeries and medications, and the raised health consciousness of the population—all factors for the good. They work longer hours, see more patients for shorter times and earn less money than they might ever have expected when they began their careers. The current health care system forces many doctors to become preoccupied with the fiscal side of medicine, which in turn cannot help but damage the trust that is essential between patients and their doctors. Another unfortunate result, exemplified by Dr. Solomon's dilemma, may be a subtle pattern of health care rationing that seems to evade public scrutiny.

One wonders whether any change in the health care system can ever fulfill our demands of medicine. Ironically, when a vast number of Americans lack basic health care, consumers today ask more and more of the system. The simple ideal of providing the best possible care to all, which drove health care at Beth Israel, the Deaconess and other hospitals during health care's "golden age," seems to have been replaced by a widespread expectation that our doctors grant us immortality.

Chapter Seven

Et Tu, Brutus?

"A truth that's told with bad intent
beats all the lies you can invent."
—William Blake

Boston's titans in medicine and health care are the large, Harvard teaching hospitals: Beth Israel Deaconess, Massachusetts General, Brigham and Women's, and Children's Hospital display a dynamic slate of brilliant researchers with reputations for providing top-quality health care, and consistently high-performing clinical, educational and administrative departments characterize each one. Like the mythological Titans, these hospitals have traditionally competed, clashed and allied on a grand scale, each striving to become and remain Boston's wealthiest and most prestigious purveyor of cutting-edge research and patient care.

By the mid-1990s even they faced a new health care system that was no longer solely driven by patient need and available treatment but, increasingly, by fiscal demands. Third-party payers were now capping reimbursements to hospitals while costs continued to rise. Hospitals had no choice but to pay the prices set by pharmaceutical and biomedical companies, insurers and private suppliers but were also faced with the growing and costly challenge of recruiting and retaining clinical staff. Operating under new mandates, Medicare and Medicaid now limited patient hospital stays and treatment. When a patient received treatment that cost more than the allowable amount, the hospitals had to bear the cost. With reimbursements inadequate to cover the cost of health care for uninsured and underinsured patients, hospitals were hemorrhaging money and many sank deeply into debt. Despite the advantageous malpractice rates provided by CRICO, the Harvard hospitals factored in malpractice insurance as a significant expense. No matter how prestigious an institution, its administration worried about remaining solvent.

HMOs, by now the health care payers and providers for large segments of the population, faced many of the same fiscal pressures that plagued the hospitals. To contain costs and ensure profitability, they began to aggressively, preferentially enroll healthy, young families. This strategy denied HMO coverage to many poor and elderly who then had to forego care or seek treatment in a hospital emergency room, for which the hospital often had to absorb the cost. This strategy initially worked well for the HMOs. However, even they began to cave in under the staggering medical costs. Harvard Pilgrim Health Plan had become one of the largest HMOs in New England and despite careful patient recruitment and aggressive mergers with other regional HMOs, Harvard Pilgrim began to falter. As the HMO reduced its payments to hospitals, the entire local health care industry suffered and in 1999, with losses well over a million dollars, Harvard Pilgrim lost its accreditation.

Some large, heavily endowed institutions had the resources to take proactive measures. Taking their cues from the banking and telecommunication industries, many merged with other institutions—a powerful and immediate way to increase market share. Mergers also brought economies of scale that reduced operational redundancies, increased buying power and bargained leverage with pharmaceutical companies, other suppliers and insurers including the federal government. The nationwide acceleration of "merger mania" caught many smaller hospitals off guard. Some were absorbed into larger institutions; others adapted their missions to fit niche markets; and still others closed their doors, often abandoning populations that had depended upon their services. For example, the venerable Cleveland Clinic closed its emergency room and refocused its resources on affluent cardiac patients.

The Harvard teaching hospitals had always vied for top researchers, clinicians, administrators, funding and patients. Now the stakes were even higher. Every health care provider's survival depended on its ability to expand market share and contain costs. The challenge demanded aggressive business maneuvering. However, few of Boston's esteemed hospital administrators were prepared to address strategic business issues such as market share, cost-efficiency and restructuring options. Most of the leaders of Harvard teaching hospitals had been trained as physicians and earned their positions through their lifelong focus on health care objectives, not an aptitude for business, accounting or law.

In 1994, with the alliance of Massachusetts General and

Brigham and Women's hospitals as Partners HealthCare, health care in Boston truly became a corporate battleground, and medical administration became a contact sport. Each "player" brought his own agenda, brilliance, strengths, ego and professional frailties. Planned and executed in secrecy, the alliance rocked the foundations of trust in the entire Boston health care community and torpedoed an effort by Dr. Daniel C. Tosteson, then Dean of Harvard Medical School, to bring the Harvard hospitals under a single canopy to facilitate collaboration. Everyone was blindsided by the announcement of the Partners alliance, from front-desk reception staff to hospital presidents and the Dean himself.

As a single, mammoth entity, Partners immediately began to leverage its might to stabilize the fiscal health of its two flagship hospitals. Starting in 1994, its strategic moves to cut costs and build market share for MGH and Brigham catalyzed a mad scramble for footing among the other hospitals. Ultimately, in 1996, the Beth Israel and Deaconess hospitals were forced to make a complicated, tension-riddled merger under a new parent corporation—CareGroup Healthcare System.

Newspaper reports, public documents and first-person accounts have helped this author create a narrative of the tumultuous events that led to the MGH-Brigham alliance. Many have written and spoken about the creation of Partners and its impact on other local hospitals and health care delivery in Boston. An axe to grind, actions to defend, individual self-interest, bias or institutional loyalty informs every version of the tale. As a result, writing a definitive narrative of the alliance between MGH and Brigham is as complicated as trying to teach a five-year-old child to read *Ulysses* in Latin.

Akira Kurosawa's 1950 film *Rashomon* demonstrated how perceptions of a single event could vary so vastly as to forever bury the truth. The story revolves around an ambush in the woods, the rape of a Japanese woman and the violent death of her husband—a suicide or a murder? Four men, each of whom observed the event, give differing accounts with tempting correlations. Yet all the accounts contain discrepancies, proving the inability of any one person to really know the objective truth no matter how clearly one thinks he or she can see it. Truth is relative and subjective and can be shaped, consciously or unconsciously, by one's personal preconceptions and motivations. As in *Rashomon*, the truth about the MGH-Brigham alliance ultimately depends on the eye of the beholder.

Ironically, it seems that Dr. Tosteson may have unwittingly sparked the alliance between Massachusetts General and Brigham. He convened all of the Harvard teaching hospitals for a very different purpose. He had grown concerned that the deepening financial crisis in health care would corrode the training, research opportunities and prestige available to an entire generation of medical students. Harvard depended on its relationships with the state-of-the-art medical centers to engage its students in high-quality research, education and patient care. Therefore the Dean was also invested in the hospitals' fiscal vitality. Dr. Tosteson invited leaders of the five Harvard teaching hospitals—Beth Israel, Deaconess, Massachusetts General, Brigham and Children's Hospital—to explore common solutions to their shared problems.

The Dean envisioned a collaboration that would enable the hospitals to market themselves efficiently, help each hospital contain costs and enhance their collective teaching and research capacity. He hoped to engage the hospitals' leaders in reducing both the duplication of services and the historically intense inter-hospital competition. He proposed that representatives of the five institutions meet regularly to discuss shared concerns and form strategies so as to operate as a single power base. He assured the institutions that their autonomy would prevail and promised that Harvard would not interfere in their operations.

The Harvard Planning Group met on January 5, 1993 as a committee of fifteen, which included the board chair, the chief executive and a prominent physician from each of the institutions. Aware that each hospital zealously guarded its independence, traditions and turf, Dr. Tosteson knew that his goals could only be achieved by gentle persuasion. He was the one player who saw the big picture and eschewed allegiance to any particular hospital. Warning the group that change was coming, he charged them with developing a new structure for managing the significant challenges inherent in financing medical care while sustaining the teaching and scholarly functions of the medical school.

Shortly after they began the monthly meetings of the Harvard Planning Group, they became mired in personal and institutional conflicts that took a fiercely competitive tone. Disturbed by the animosity and mistrust, Dr. Tosteson sought feedback from Dr. Samuel Thier, then president of Brandeis University and later president of Partners HealthCare. Dr. Thier replied, "You'll be lucky if you get two to agree. They don't trust what you're doing." Some participants feared that Massachusetts General, the largest non-governmental employer in Boston with more than 5,000 physicians, nurses and maintenance and housekeeping employees, would dominate a consortium. Others raised concerns about antitrust issues or expressed the desire to maintain the status quo. One participant told Dr. Tosteson that he had not heard anything compelling or important enough to move them toward collaboration.

Subsequently, Dr. Tosteson learned that some participants had suspected him of a hidden agenda to gain control over the hospitals. Outside observers simply thought the proposed consortium was too unwieldy. David Bray, then Dean of administration of Harvard (a position subsequently held by Paul Levy, now president of Beth Israel Deaconess Medical Center), told an associate that he thought the sheer size of the Harvard Planning Group—five large hospitals—would impede widespread reform. Of Dr. Tosteson, Mr. Bray said, "His captain's ship was very large and consequently could only turn slowly."

Because the hospitals were not officially accountable to Harvard, the Dean could not mandate collaboration. Yet his hopes sustained his effort. Despite the contentious, artificial tone of the June 14, 1993 meeting, which he recalled ten years later as frustrating, he was pleased when the participants agreed on that date to work together as one overall entity. Dean Tosteson began writing a proposal to form the Harvard Medical Group. With signatures from all five hospitals, the proposal would become a plan for collaboration.

After that meeting, as some of the members headed off to lunch, Dr. Robert Buchanan, CEO of Massachusetts General, was overheard saying to MGH board president Ferdinand Colloredo-Mansfield and Dean John McArthur of Harvard Business School, "These meetings would be really energized if we and the Brigham got together"; and then, "We should do it ourselves. The Dean's plan would never work." Within forty-eight hours, the Massachusetts General Hospital leadership had made an agreement with Dr. Richard Nesson, CEO of Brigham, to withdraw from Dr. Tosteson's planning group and explore strategies on their own. The MGH and Brigham leadership agreed they would not commit their institution to joining the Dean's proposed consortium.

A few days later Dean McArthur and Mr. Francis "Hooks" Burr, an attorney and MGH trustee, told Dr. Tosteson that MGH would no longer participate in either the meetings or the proposed consortium. However, they assured him, MGH and Brigham representatives would regularly report the progress of their bilateral discussions to the Dean. In fact, the plans for a formal MGH-Brigham affiliation had already begun in ironclad privacy, as advised by the management-consulting firm Boston Consulting Group. Neither hospital honored the promise that Mr. Burr and Dean McArthur had made to keep the Dean informed.

In 2003 a third person recalled Dean McArthur telling colleagues that the force driving the Partners alliance was the potential power of the combined hospitals to influence, if not dominate, the regional health care market. Further, Dean McArthur knew that speed was essential to the impact of the alliance. "We will do a case study of the alliance, give ourselves from July Fourth to Thanksgiving to write the case study, then sell it during the next week," he told a colleague. A very small inner circle safeguarded the plan; however, when Massachusetts General's chief of surgery, Dr. Gerald Austin, expressed his discomfort about withholding information from his staff, he was given permission to share information.

MGH and Brigham successfully pulled a shroud of secrecy over their plans that rivaled that of Hillary Clinton's health care task force. By the end of 1993, the management of the two hospitals had formulated a plan to ally as Partners Health Care, Inc. This massive entity would absorb a number of smaller institutions, force restructuring at still others and buy out dozens of private physician practices. Representatives of the remaining three Harvard teaching hospitals—Beth Israel, Deaconess and Children's—continued to meet with Dean Tosteson. Unaware of the alliance, they assumed they were working on a plan that encompassed the entire group.

The two hospitals announced the Partners alliance at a Sunday morning press conference on December 6, 1993, catching not only the general public off guard but also Dr. Tosteson, the staffs of both MGH and Brigham, *Boston Globe* reporters and Dr. Mitchell Rabkin, then president of Beth Israel Hospital. As a senior member of Dean Tosteson's Harvard Planning Group, Dr. Rabkin had looked forward to sharing the communal expertise and wisdom to address the health care financial crisis. In 2003 he recalled that he had been in Israel when told by a reporter the news of the MGH-Brigham alliance. He said he'd thought a more appropriate time for the announcement would have been December 7, the day Pearl Harbor had been attacked in 1941. His dismay, shock and anger were eminently apparent.

Awaiting him in Boston were monumental pressures and concerns about the survival of the remaining hospitals. At that time, when hospitals were in dire financial straits and the new Goliath was fully armed, medical institutions were truly in jeopardy. Partners had created a situation that was a polar opposite of the Dean's intentions.

Dean Tosteson learned of the MGH-Brigham alliance while

attending a conference at Boston's World Trade Center, moments before First Lady Hillary Clinton was to speak on health care reform. A Harvard faculty member attending the meeting told Dean Tosteson he'd heard a rumor that a deal had been cut. Later that day, Mr. Burr, attorney for the MGH and Dean McArthur, personally informed him of the Partners alliance. Stunned but gracious, Dr. Tosteson congratulated them and called it a great achievement. The Dean immediately reported the news to Harvard president Neil Rudenstein and learned that MGH and Brigham trustees had already informed him of their alliance. In 2003 Dr. Tosteson recalled his sadness not only because he had been kept utterly in the dark about Partners' formation but also because one of his most prestigious teaching hospitals had completely bypassed his office in publicizing the news.

Inevitably, the covert alliance sparked feelings of betrayal throughout the medical community, especially at Harvard Medical School and the other teaching hospitals. The ability of MGH and Brigham to conceal their plans from the Dean, Dr. Rabkin and their peers exemplified the lack of honesty with which these men operated. All were experts in medicine and hospital administration but few had sophisticated mastery of finance, strategic planning or mergers and acquisitions. Though cognizant of interinstitutional rivalry, no one in the medical community would have imagined that a peer institution would make a move that so threatened the survival of so many renowned, venerable institutions. The leaders of all regional medical institutions had been blindsided.

Almost immediately the new executive management team and advisory board took on the leadership of Partners HealthCare, created a new logo and advertised on the Web sites of MGH and Brigham. The lay public assumed this was a merged institution. In fact, the two hospitals had not merged, only allied. Affiliation, as opposed to merging, was Partners' brilliant decision. The two hospitals immediately gained the ability to cut their expenses through advantageous contracts with insurers, pharmaceutical firms and other suppliers while avoiding the complexity of a true merger. By integrating backroom operations including accounting, purchasing and billing, the two hospitals consolidated their administrative tasks and costs and facilitated purchasing supplies in bulk. However, MGH and Brigham did not integrate their clinical departments except for surgery and orthopedics. Health care services and funded research continued as usual. Chiefs of service, clinical department heads and staff retained their existing positions at each institution. The hospitals' trustees remained members of their respective boards except for those trustees who were hand-picked to join the new Partners' advisory board.

The alliance diffused a longstanding competition between MGH and Brigham. Dr. David Blumenthal, an authority on health care management, said that by the time of the alliance, the two were each other's principal competition. Dr. Richard Nesson, the CEO who left Brigham to become CEO of Partners, noted that they had always been competitive when it came to attracting the best students and residents in addition to renowned surgeons. Before the alliance, MGH had been cast as the complacent king, and Brigham was the upstart that threatened to displace it.

Outsiders viewed the senior clinical staff as "clubby." Compared with Brigham, MGH was a more self-assured institution and was quite comfortable disagreeing with Harvard. Dr. Roger Lange, a Beth Israel oncologist and hematologist, said, "MGH was always threatening to pull out of the medical school completely and start their own medical school. They asked, 'Why do we need Harvard Medical School?'" In his 2001 study of teaching-hospital mergers, Dr. Kastor said, "MGH's territorial pride was a deep institutional trait that would have been a continuing obstacle to a more complete integration."

A variety of additional factors would have made merging MGH and Brigham and Women's clinical services extremely difficult. Brigham was resident-run, with faculty surgeons rotating on-and-off service. Faculty physicians at MGH retained greater control over their patients' treatments. In a 2002 *New York Times* article, "Merged Hospitals Gain Both Power and Critics," Reed Abelson reported that Partners' CEO, Dr. James J. Mongan, voiced the opinion that a merger of MGH and Brigham would never have made sense "given their locations and other factors: a twenty-minute drive from each other." By allying instead of merging, MGH and Brigham solved their respective fiscal problems without compromising the culture or efficiency of either institution.

In the same 2002 *New York Times* story, Dr. Mongan attributed $250 million in cost savings to the alliance. However, the story noted that these savings would not be funneled into cost reductions for consumers but instead would increase Partners' coffers. Beneficial as it was for its two principal hospitals, Partners' powerful forward motion caused repercussions throughout the regional health care system. The fiscal efficiency of the MGH-Brigham alliance tightened the squeeze on the other Harvard teaching hospitals. As the Partners' hospitals consolidated their costs and garnered greater market share, they automatically improved their fiscal performance in contrast to the other hospitals and cut into the others' market share. In his 2002 article, Mr. Abelson quoted Dr. David Mulligan, a former Massachusetts public health physician: "The alliance made health care here more expensive and weakened the local institutions."

Partners moved aggressively to increase its income, cut costs and dominate the region's health care. By initiating exclusive relationships with small, community hospitals and private physician practices, Partners spread across the region, intensifying the other Harvard teaching hospitals' struggles to maintain, if not expand, market share. Partners' push for higher and quicker payments from HMOs has been well documented. At one point, Partners announced that it would apply for a license to create its own HMO if existing insurers did not pay in a timely manner. What HMOs and other non-governmental health plans pay hospitals was unknown. However, the Partners hospitals' revenue from inpatient services as reported to the Commonwealth of Massachusetts rose twenty-six percent from 1996 to 2001, while comparable institutions' inpatient revenue rose just sixteen percent.

Within a few years, Partners announced its intent to build a large, outpatient, primary-care center in the Fresh Pond section of Cambridge. This facility would have actively competed with Mt. Auburn Hospital, a highly respected community hospital that became affiliated with CareGroup Healthcare System. Partners readily attracted patients from the surrounding towns of Waltham, Belmont, Watertown and Cambridge. Was Partners simply blustering? The competing facility in Cambridge never came to fruition but such a move would have significantly damaged Mt. Auburn Hospital's census. According to a staff physician then working at Mt. Auburn Hospital, Partners threatened to take all of the specialty-care patients being served at the smaller hospital, and that anyone who needed cardiac surgery would go to MGH.

To this day Partners continues to cause significant problems for management of all area hospitals. In January 2006 *The Boston Globe* reported, "Partners Health Care is using market clout to pressure a North Shore hospital group and its three hundred doctors, who were losing money, to send their patients to Partners' facilities in Salem, Massachusetts." Northeast Health's physicians had angered Partners management by referring advanced-care patients to North Shore hospitals outside the Partners network. Partners threatened to exclude Northeast Health System from their group. Six months later columnist Steve Bailey wrote in *The Boston Globe,* "Northeast will lose lucrative affiliation agreements unless it cooperates more fully in Partners' vision for a health care network." According to the *Globe*, Partners' threat represented a personal income cut of ten to twenty percent for each physician affiliated with Northeast Health. Some months later, the announcement of a Partners plan to open a $100-million outpatient facility in the neighboring town of Danvers, Massachusetts, was turning up the heat on Northeast Health Systems still more.

Partners claimed that its in-network restrictions served patients by ensuring their access to prime clinical care. *The Boston Globe* quoted an alternate view from Mr. Paul Levy, CEO of CareGroup and BIDMC: "This is a heavy handed assault on high quality, independent hospitals...part of a clearly conceived plan by Partners to obtain even more market dominance in the North Shore region." The *Globe* further suggested that Partners' actions constituted financial inducements to physicians for patient referrals, a practice prohibited under federal law.

In November 2006 *Boston Globe* columnist Bailey wrote, "Thirteen years after Harvard Business School's Dean John McArthur, Mr. Ferdinando Collerado-Mansfield, and others combined Massachusetts' best brand names in health care, it is clear the merger is working for Partners. What is unclear after all this time is whether it is working for anyone else."

Partners and Blue Cross/Blue Shield were hosting a conference on regional health care collaboration while simultaneously refusing to cooperatively share an expensive, suburban cancer radiation facility with other area hospitals. Steve Bailey's column called attention to the irony this exposed. In 2004 Beth Israel Deaconess Medical Center approached Partners with an offer to share and, if necessary, move its underutilized radiation center from Waltham to Partners' Newton Wellesley Hospital. Partners refused the offer and began the process of building itself a similar facility for $13.2 million in Newton, an adjacent town.

Mr. Paul Levy told *The Boston Globe*, "This seemed to be a clear case of where two hospitals could share and optimize the use of an expensive facility to benefit the public and both hospitals. Basically we were turned down." Newton Wellesley Hospital's president, Dr. Michael Jellinek, rejected aspects of Mr. Levy's offer and Dr. Mongan offered this consolation: "Society itself is conflicted about when it wants nonprofits to collaborate and when to compete."

Not surprisingly, the 2006 Partners-hosted conference "was

more than they could swallow," wrote Steve Bailey of Mr. Levy and Charles Baker, CEO of Harvard Pilgrim Health Care, "Here was Partners—the Coke and Pepsi of the state's hospital industry—preaching the gospel of collaboration. This from an organization that has grown so large and rich that it has essentially defined the market as Partners and Everyone Else."

Besides enduring, with the other Harvard teaching hospitals, the challenges of facing Goliath, Beth Israel Hospital suffered directly from Partners' business actions. Early on, Dr. Michael Zinner, chief of surgery at Brigham, set the stage for ensuing battles for market share with the remark, "Everyone not with you is a competitor." In retrospect one can see many of Partners' actions as simple though perhaps unduly cold business maneuvers. However, many Beth Israel senior staff members continue to believe that Partners, from its inception, targeted their hospital for annihilation. "Big guns were trained on the hospital and we were caught in the crosshairs," said one former Beth Israel administrator in 2003. "The Beth Israel was a target for destruction. They wanted to kill Mitch Rabkin," said another former administrator. Dr. Lange, an oncologist, cited several times when Partners took aim at Beth Israel: "They undercut us with Harvard Community Health Plan. The Brigham gave away beds at low or no cost, enticing patients away from the Beth Israel."

Some interviewees said that Partners continued "to display animosity and overt aggression toward the Beth Israel even after the Beth Israel-Deaconess merger." Dr. Kim Saal, a cardiologist at Beth Israel Hospital, said that for a decade, Partners perceived Beth

Israel as a threat. As the financial recovery of Beth Israel Deaconess Medical Center gathered speed in 2000, Dr. Saal said Partners "tried to stunt their growth."

Dr. Rabkin lacked the training or the conscience to respond to Partners' actions with the swift aggression needed to protect the multimillion-dollar corporation his hospital had become. As a businessman, he was no match for those steering the Partners alliance. However, in addition to the business problems, Dr. Rabkin became Dr. Richard Nesson's personal target. Having previously been Beth Israel colleagues and friends for many years, Dr. Nesson suddenly became an antagonist.

"When Dr. Nesson became CEO of the Brigham, he developed an inordinately hostile, competitive attitude toward Mitch and the Beth Israel," recalled Dr. Jack Kasten, who had maintained a friendship with both men over decades. In the mid-1990s, with the might of the Partners behind him, Dr. Nesson escalated his attacks on Beth Israel and on Dr. Rabkin himself. He played a key role in the recruitment of Dr. Eugene Brawnwald as chief of medicine and is known to be one of the most able administrators in the field of academic medicine. For nine years, Dr. Braunwald held a joint appointment at Beth Israel and Brigham and Women's, an arrangement approved by Dr. Nesson and Dr. Rabkin. Dr. Braunwald chaired both hospitals' departments of medicine and under his leadership both flourished. Not long after the Partners alliance was in operation, Dr. Braunwald was prevailed upon to leave Beth Israel and accept a key administrative position with Partners.

There is little question that Dr. Nesson's behavior negatively affected Beth Israel's senior staff and exacerbated the problems confronting Dr. Rabkin. Former senior staff recalled being perplexed by Dr. Nesson's anger. Though the animosity was common knowledge in the Harvard medical community, no one has offered a definitive explanation. However, there's little question that Dr. Nesson's behavior negatively affected Beth Israel senior staff.

Dr. Lange offered another perspective, saying that Dr. Nesson left Beth Israel shortly after Dr. Howard Hiatt, a highly esteemed, nationally known physician, left Beth Israel to assume the position of CEO at Brigham. Dr. Lange said, "Dr. Nesson was Dr. Hiatt's 'hit man.' He was like a god who would ride through on a white horse, lift his finger and point to the one who had to be destroyed." Thus Dr. Hiatt's hands remained clean and Dr. Nesson "would kill the giants who required killing." Dr. Lange reflected that perhaps Dr. Nesson had been passed over for a promotion when Dr. Howard Hiatt went to Brigham. Shortly after Dr. Nesson's move to Harvard Pilgrim he followed Dr. Hiatt to Brigham. "I know no reason for his enmity toward Dr. Rabkin. It was personal," Dr. Lange said. "It could not have been anti-Semitism since they were both Jewish." Dr. Nesson had served on the Beth Israel staff for several years, yet never included this information in his *curriculum vitae*. Dr. Kasten said, "Their common interests, intellects, and professions created a close bond. When the intense, competitive behavior began, I felt bad." Dean Tosteson, when interviewed, said, "If you ever learn the cause of the animosity, please let me know."

In recent years, Partners developed a program in which MGH and Brigham specialists traveled worldwide to evaluate and treat wealthy individuals and encourage those patients to travel to Boston to continue their medical care. The alliance has expanded to include non-acute health care including rehabilitation services, nursing homes and home-care services. One such facility is a nursing home masquerading as a rehabilitation center: North End Rehabilitation Center.

In retrospect one must acknowledge that the hospitals' managers had the freedom and the right to reconfigure their institutions with accountability to no one but their trustees. Their corporate and legal skills were finely honed, their shrewdness and business acumen beyond compare. Taking a leaf from Hillary Clinton's book, they covered their activities with a blanket of secrecy. Thus they had no need to defend their alliance until it was a *fait accompli*.

Even if Dean Tosteson had been alerted to the plan, he could not have interfered. What was notably missing from the Partners alliance was the honor and respect due the Dean and their colleagues. The cut of the betrayal left a large scar across the Harvard medical community that has yet to fully heal. The nub of the issue and the source of the lingering pain caused by the Partners alliance is not what its architects did, but rather the way they did it. Mr. Paul Levy, president and CEO of CareGroup, reflected in 2003 that Partners took "the two strongest siblings in the Harvard system, left the family, and created their own." He went on to say that Dean Tosteson was "blown away when two of his affiliates would do this without telling him."

Meanwhile health care workers at Beth Israel and the other Harvard teaching hospitals absorbed the tensions and rallied to deliver patient care as usual, and continued to provide the highest-quality patient care in a work environment tainted by increasing paperwork, job insecurity, frequent new policies and procedures aimed at cutting costs, and top-level changes in clinical staffing. While no research to date has quantified the effect of staff anxiety on patient care in Boston's hospitals during the 1990s, firsthand accounts recall the dampened morale among frontline caregivers.

Like a mom-and-pop grocery store adjacent to a new Super Stop & Shop, Beth Israel continued to lose great sums of money while at the same time trying to stave off Partners. With the Massachusetts attorney general threatening Beth Israel with receivership, the hospital's leadership saw merging as its only option. A rapid succession of CEOs, six in four years, presided over a very complicated merger with Deaconess Hospital. Instability fed internal confusion, anger and conflict. Yet quality patient care was never compromised and the BIDMC remains a state-of-the-art medical center.

At this writing, Beth Israel Deaconess Medical Center and its parent company, Care Group, have rebounded financially under the leadership of Mr. Levy, with most merger-related difficulties now behind them. While Partners' business strategies continue to make more enemies than friends, the actions of Goliath are no longer secret but come under more public scrutiny than ever before.

Chapter 8

Perish or Prosper

"Live like brothers but do business as strangers."
—Anonymous

L ate in the twentieth century, many teaching hospitals nation-wide were confronted with an increasingly punitive medical climate. The Clintons' promise of "health care for all" had, in fact, done little more than illuminate the system's numerous flaws and diminish hopes for national reform. Although costs continued to rise, insurance companies reduced reimbursements. Many malpractice insurers abandoned unprofitable markets, including Massachusetts. Though CRICO (Controlled Risk Insurance Company) formed in the 1970s and continued to exclusively insure Harvard-affiliated hospitals and physicians, but the government withdrew support for medical student education. Fiscally, it was impossible for medical centers to survive as standalone institutions and continue to excel at research, teaching and patient care. Attempting to balance both components was onerous and represented the plight of hospitals throughout the country.

Jack Kasden, Beth Israel Hospital administrator, admonished his colleagues: "A hospital is not a business but should be run as one." He recognized the duality of medicine as a business and a craft, with both components essential to a hospital's fiscal solvency and its ability to provide uncompromising health care.

Primed for a change and without any public notice, two hospitals took it upon themselves to find a survival strategy and allied in 1994. Massachusetts General and Brigham and Women's hospitals were Boston's two largest Harvard teaching hospitals and they became a Goliath medical center. Well cushioned with enormous endowments, they feared no competitors. Now confronted with this powerful, new alliance, the others scurried to choose partners, preferably from among those affiliated with Harvard Medical School, Tufts New England Medical Center and Boston University's medical school. Exploratory meetings were rampant but few deals were consummated. A potential merger of Tufts-New England Medical Center and the Harvard-affiliated Deaconess hospital evaporated with the realization that the two, under the aegis of separate medical schools, could not unite and serve both masters. Two other major, inner-city institutions, Boston City Hospital and Boston University Medical Center, did merge in 1996 aided by the efforts of Boston's mayor and successful negotiations with several labor unions including the House Officer's Union. Boston City Hospital, a renowned institution, serviced Boston's indigent and socially disadvantaged. Boston University Medical Center, in close proximity to Boston City Hospital, is their primary teaching hospital.

The merger activity in Boston reflected a national trend in health care that had begun among HMOs. The 1995 merger of Harvard Community Health Plan and Pilgrim Health Plan created a managed-care health plan with approximately one million enrollees. The academic medical centers would be even more vulnerable if HMOs were, as had been suggested, transformed into for-profit entities. Over a several-year period in the 1990s, U.S. hospitals undertook 1,115 mergers to better compete and negotiate with ever-more-powerful HMOs. As hospitals merged across the nation everyone held their collective breath, waiting to see which merger would succeed. Eighty-seven of the 1,115 did not last. St. Louis' Barnes Jewish Hospital and Children's Hospital merged and are known as BJC. Some academic facilities closed. A merger of the medical institutions of Stanford University and the University of California failed within a few years but not because its purpose wasn't compelling. One of the California executives had said to the other before they'd merged, "We can't succeed with the arms race with such marginal bottom lines. We're going to kill each other if we don't find a way to work together."

To guarantee their profitability, HMOs handpicked young, healthy enrollees. The academic medical centers would be even more vulnerable if these large HMOs were, as had been suggested, transformed into for-profit entities.

Beyond the trend toward mergers, the competition for health care market share transformed into a feeding frenzy as providers of all sizes became involved in the "growth by acquisition" strategy. Big fish ate the little ones as hospitals and health plans began to include smaller facilities and private physician practices in their exclusive networks, or bought them outright. Dr. Solomon's "pod" was such a practice. In New England all of the Harvard teaching hospitals expanded their provider networks of affiliated and hospital-employed medical practitioners during the 1990s. Meanwhile smaller Harvard community hospitals and clinics closed, in some cases, after being sold to a larger health care organization.

In October 1996 the media announced that Beth Israel hospital, Pathway Health Network, Deaconess, Mount Auburn Foundation and New England Baptist hospital would merge and be among the largest networks in the Northeast. More than 10,000 employees, 1,200 active medical staff and nearly $1 billion in revenue organized to form a system of health care. The newly named Beth Israel Deaconess Medical Center (BIDMC) would encompass both hospitals' campuses in Boston's Longwood Medical area. Dr. Rabkin said, "We will become a single, streamlined entity rather than a *fatter institution*. Coming together increases our ability to offer high-quality care more efficiently and to negotiate more effectively in competing with managed care programs and other insurers." Dr. J. Richard Gaitner, chief executive of Pathway, also expressed high hopes for the merger, saying, "Collaboration will allow us to fulfill our mission and to compete effectively in today's rapidly changing market. Accordingly, the network's strength is drawn from diversity and competence of the founding institutions of Beth Israel Medical Center, Mount Auburn Hospital, the community affiliates of Pathway Health Network, and New England Baptist and the excellence of their associated physicians."

A key local feature of this rapidly changing market was the Partners alliance, by then a $1.8-billion network including MGH, Brigham and Women's, McLean Hospital, Spaulding Rehabilitation Hospital and many smaller facilities.

In 2003 several Beth Israel and Deaconess participants in the merger were asked whether they had considered replicating the Partners alliance rather than merging. Under the Partners umbrella, the presidents of MGH and Brigham had continued to captain their own ships and managed their respective domains the day after the alliance, just as they had done the day before. By 1996 Partners had trimmed operating costs, built a healthy profit margin, gained market share and attracted new staff while preserving each flagship hospital's trustees, CEOs and staff. Why had Beth Israel not followed the model of the alliance? Beth Israel and Deaconess administration unanimously responded that they had never considered it as an option. Dr. Rabkin reiterated what he'd said at the time: "We had agreed to merge and were going to do a true merger, combining functions, assets, consolidation of clinical departments and staff with one president and a single board of trustees." Governance would provide economies of fiscal scale while enhancing the quality of health care provided to patients. They would then be a player in reshaping Boston's health care industry. Theirs was a philosophy of promoting long life and well-being and their mission was to create a value-driven, price-competitive, regional-integrated delivery system with a network that would provide a full array of superior health care services to outpatients and communities. The system was to be restructured with a single board derived from the merged entities and it was to be an integrated system of community-based primary-care physicians with hospitals and health care centers serving communities in eastern Massachusetts. He hoped it would be a template for successful mergers throughout the country.

Dean Daniel Tosteson of Harvard Medical School noted that

each institution's faculty participated enthusiastically in the design of Harvard Medical School's new Pathways for General Medical Education system, which was structured under a single board derived from the merged parent entities. Mount Auburn and New England Baptist hospital would continue as two distinct hospitals under BIDMC's umbrella and would have meaningful representation in the merged parent company. Mr. Francis P. Lynch, then president of Mount Auburn, said that they chose to merge with BIDMC due to its ongoing commitment to community-based medicine.

Dr. John Kastor's 2001 study analyzed the mergers of teaching hospitals and catalogued the potential benefits of merging. Yet he noted that, in many cases, the board members who devised these combinations underestimated how difficult it would be to unite administrators, doctors, nurses and trustees from institutions that were incredibly diverse. The Beth Israel and Deaconess merger is a case in point. It did succeed in keeping the merged institutions afloat in the unforgiving managed-care market but from the outset, the hospital's two cultures collided: Jewish versus Methodist, consensus versus corporate-style decision making, general medical care versus specialty care.

Similar philosophies between the two hospitals encouraged optimism for the merger. Both shared an affiliation with Harvard Medical School and a triple mission of patient care, medical education and research. Clinical expertise and respect for individuals were the underlying philosophies of each hospital and each retained their religious roots. Each hospital's legacy included a cadre of devoted, talented, volunteer women who made major contributions to the hospital's growth and development, and they had a dedicated community of trustees and donors.

The merger magnified significant differences between Beth Israel and Deaconess staff. In retrospect, many administrators, trustees and staff involved with the merger felt as though due diligence had been inadequate on both sides. The merger was akin to a hastily formed marriage between two parties who hardly knew each other. From the start, clashes best described as "cultures" seriously disturbed the work environment of BIDMC including senior management, clinical chiefs of service, physicians, nurses and trustees. Adding fuel to the fire, Beth Israel's senior managers, president and board chair were placed in power over their Deaconess counterparts. Acrimony was inevitable.

The issues seemed to defy tolerable solutions. How does an organization remove one of two highly esteemed hospital presidents? How does a newly formed management team amalgamate two medical staffs, both rich with expertise? Combining two boards of trustees seemed impossible. How could fruitful discussion or a vote be accomplished when as many as fifty dedicated, well-qualified people wanted a role in shaping the hospital's agenda? Dr. Kastor described the Beth Israel-Deaconess merger as a "true merger of assets and function."

CareGroup forced together the clinical departments in both Harvard teaching hospitals under single chiefs. All but one were Beth Israel appointments. Though described by its designers as a merger of equals, many perceived the formation as a takeover of the Deaconess by Beth Israel. Dr. Rabkin, then president of Beth Israel, became CareGroup's president while Deaconess president

Dr. Gaitner became second in command. Mr. Stephen Kaye, chairman of Beth Israel, chaired the combined board while Pathway's chairman, John Hamill, assumed the role of vice chair.

Should one have expected some magnanimity in the selection of chiefs with some positions granted to chiefs from each hospital? The existing chiefs in both hospitals were well qualified to head a merged department yet the only remaining Deaconess chief was Dr. Andrew Brotman, chief of psychiatry. The demotion of so many Deaconess chiefs rapidly led to staff departures.

Upon hearing of the merger, the anesthesiology department left the Deaconess. While the Beth Israel anesthesiologists were salaried hospital employees, the Deaconess department of anesthesiology was an independent service not on the hospital's payroll. In fact they paid the Deaconess for the use of its operating rooms and retained the income paid for the services they provided. In addition they had contracts with numerous suburban hospitals and were referred to as "itinerant anesthesiologists." Prior to their departure they adopted silo behavior, meaning they retreated into their own space and avoided collegial exchange and engagement.

Simply said, there can be no surgery without anesthesia. Following their departure, Dr. Roger Jenkins, chief of transplant surgery, moved his twenty-eight-member team from BIDMC to Lahey Clinic. Interviewed in 2006, Dr. Ronald Weintraub, chief of surgery emeritus at Beth Israel, suggested that some rancor might have been averted had BIDMC allowed transplant surgery to be done at the Deaconess and cardiac surgery at Beth Israel. This plan would have provided each group a measure of independence and a sense of having their own turf. Instead, BIDMC incurred a financial loss of approximately $20,000 per liver transplant. With morale already at a low ebb, some administrators, doctors and staff nurses left Care Group, thereby disrupting its functioning, diminishing its capacity and adding to major fiscal losses. Dr. Gaitner, president emeritus of the Deaconess, remained one year post-merger, then left to assume the presidency of a Southern hospital.

The Beth Israel and Deaconess hospitals—Pathway Health Network—sought their survival strategy by completely merging on April 25, 1996. For several weeks prior, they held exploratory discussions. The outcome under consideration would include con- solidation of clinical departments, administrative functions and governance along with substantial reduction of fixed costs. This would create economies of intellectual and fiscal scale while enhanc- ing both quality and efficiency of performance and service.

Dr. Mitchell Rabkin said, "This cooperative relationship would help the community physicians to stay at the leading edge of medi- cal knowledge, diagnosis, and treatment while keeping the medical center physicians in touch with and supportive of the needs of the people in their local communities and their local physicians."

John Hamill, Pathway's board chair, hailed the joining of these two major Harvard-affiliated teaching hospitals as "permitting the vital changes in economics and clinical programs that will provide patients, their physicians, and their health plans with sophisticated medical care, a geographically diverse network of primary-care providers and the exceptional qualities of service and care for which Beth Israel and Deaconess are justifiably renowned." The new network of hospitals, physicians and other health professionals throughout the region would include the Pathway Health Network institutions in addition to Deaconess Hospital—New England Baptist Hospital, Deaconess-Glover Hospital, Deaconess-Nashoba

Hospital and now Deaconess-Waltham—and their physicians as well as many groups of community physicians related to the Beth Israel.

The more formal phase of discussions, involving due diligence with detailed sharing of information and knowledge about the participants, lasted several months.

Joyce Clifford said the Deaconess trustees were much more vocal at board meetings than the Beth Israel members, who offered no challenges. She also said that she felt a sense of betrayal when it came to the behavior of her own trustees and that it seemed as though Deaconess agendas were always put ahead of other issues. All the while, the Beth Israel board members remained inordinately silent and unsupportive of the senior management team. Clearly, the restructuring of both boards did not produce the positive results that would propel the group toward a single purpose.

Dr. Rabkin's several decades of unquestionably effective leadership appeared to begin falling apart in 1994. Understandably he and his management team were stunned by the MGH-Brigham Partners alliance. Dr. Rabkin, Joyce Clifford and the entire Beth Israel management team appeared immobilized and unsure of a way to create a viable plan for the next generation. Rather than aggressively seeking corporate strategies, they maintained their integrity and stood fast to their earlier ways of operating. The administration of the "hospital with a heart" seemed to balk at any modification that might possibly threaten the perfection they believed they had achieved at Beth Israel. It was as though the hospital's identity was a Faberge egg that would shatter if touched. Though understandable and perhaps admirable, his regard for the people and the processes that defined Beth Israel did not help Dr. Rabkin maneuver in the post-Partners market or manage the merger with the Deaconess.

By definition, leadership is a multifaceted concept that embodies authority, power, guidance and benevolence. A leader whose style emphasizes mentorship and consensus can certainly set and achieve goals. He or she may also excel in providing a work climate that fosters productivity, creativity and self-esteem, as Dr. Rabkin surely had in the 1970s and 1980s. He and Joyce Clifford, chief of nursing, had worked together for decades and built what many considered to be a model hospital.

However the changes in the health care system and negative events in the local and national medical environment stymied them. Problem solving by consensus could no longer be an effective mechanism for decision making in a climate that required rapid response to highly complicated decisions and that all involved had an equal voice.

Restructuring and refocusing the boards of trustees was a necessary step in a good-faith effort to totally merge two hospitals. The administrators saw no alternative. Mr. Kaye believed that Beth Israel had to find a partner or else go under. Regretably, the due diligence process that preceded the merger failed to adequately identify cultural, social and even religious differences between the two boards that would, after the merger, feed conflict among BIDMC trustees and thus contribute to the hospital's accumulation of red ink. The Deaconess board members said that Beth Israel took over their hospital. Some claimed that Beth Israel trustees sought to achieve a measure of social acceptance through relationships with Deaconess trustees. Did the Beth Israel trustees find their Deaconess counterparts a more socially desirable group? Was anti-Semitism a *sub rosa* issue? When interviewed in 2003, a senior Beth Israel trustee was pleased to say that after the merger he socialized with Deaconess trustees. Now he plays golf at The Country Club in Brookline, a place from which Jews had previously been barred.

One of the most contentious areas of conflict was between the nursing staffs of both hospitals. Deaconess nurses felt as though the Beth Israel nurses were dismissive of them. According to the Deaconess nurses, Beth Israel nurses thought themselves better trained, earned higher salaries and were highly empowered to make decisions for their patients. Nurses in each group thought of themselves as the better nurses. There was a major difference. Beth Israel nurses trained in the primary nursing model and were indeed empowered to make decisions on behalf of their patients. Deaconess nurses took directions from the physicians. Beth Israel nurses' relationships with physicians were collegial, not subordinate, and they could challenge a physician's order if they thought differently about a course of treatment. These collegial relationships were a longstanding aspect of the Beth Israel culture where nurses, for decades, had benefited from expert instruction and had the respect of Harvard-affiliated physicians. The Deaconess had become a Harvard teaching hospital in 1970 and maintained more traditional doctor-nurse working relationships, which did not promote collegiality.

In many ways, the Beth Israel staff resembled children devoted to their father, as he was to them. In interviews with Beth Israel's former senior vice presidents, it was clear that they loved, admired and trusted Dr. Rabkin. Their dedication and loyalty to Beth Israel over many years was really a reflection of their loyalty to him. One member of the management team compared Dr. Rabkin's situation at Beth Israel in the mid-1990s to that of a parent who becomes less open to younger, creative thinking. Some might then become authoritative, less flexible and wed to the past. In a hospital leader, this implies a diminished capacity for strategic growth and change. A former Deaconess board member who refused to be tape recorded or identified for this book said that the merger may have gone more smoothly if Dr. Rabkin had been more flexible and willing to reshape his original conception of the Beth Israel "family." As it was, Dr. Rabkin, it seemed, was standing in the way of progress. Due diligence was inadequate on both sides and many complicated issues were not sufficiently, carefully thought through.

Even prior to the merger, Beth Israel nurses had begun to mourn the connections they had previously been able to establish with patients. Shorter in-hospital stays accounted for some. Managed health care's restrictions and cost-cutting measures placed more and more constraints on the nurses' jobs. The rewarding opportunities to offer personal attention to patients had become less frequent. In 1996 nursing at Beth Israel became less gratifying in yet another way as the merger brought disruptions and tension into the workday. The merger would not include layoffs of nurses, an anathema to the Beth Israel Deaconess. Instead they would rely on attrition to trim staff. The BIDMC continued to support Joyce Clifford's primary nursing model and her academic institutes. Yet the dissonant, hostile atmosphere in the newly merged nursing department led to departures. Trish Gibbons, a senior nurse manager, had participated in the development of the primary nursing program at Beth Israel and left to work for Partners HealthCare. Seven senior nurses and nurse managers also left the hospital. This was a major loss.

In retrospect it appears that if Dr. Rabkin's closest and most loyal advisors had been more forthright with him and shared their thinking, the outcome might have been different. In the years between the Partners formation and Dr. Rabkin's stepping down, Beth Israel's senior management withheld telling truth to power for fear of wounding him. They saw him as needing protection from Partners and the internal fiscal problems that threatened Beth Israel's survival. Though their intentions and efforts were generated by kindness, they experienced a crisis of conscience that helped bring down their beloved leader. When he stepped down, some said the Beth Israel lost its soul. One vice president said the hospital was like a huge jigsaw puzzle and he knew where all the pieces fit.

Beyond the many ways in which the newly merged staff were at odds, BIDMC was also confronted with staggering financial problems and government-mandated, intense competition from larger medical facilities. It was evident that they could no longer function as a small, family-owned business. It was, in fact, a multimillion-dollar corporation.

Before the merger, Beth Israel Deaconess shared detailed information about their respective arrangements with affiliated providers in a due diligence process that lasted for several months. However, little preparation had been made for the underperforming subsidiaries. At the time of the merger, CareGroup owned the five community hospitals that belonged to the Deaconess parent corporation, Pathway, as well as the hospitals and providers owned by Beth Israel. Few were producing the desired income. The combined losses were now a shared obligation for all CareGroup management. In 1996 animosity was engendered when CareGroup required the profitable New England Baptist and Mount Auburn hospitals to subsidize the institution's corporate losses.

Deaconess Pathway had purchased community hospitals in Waltham, Glover, Nashoba and Needham along with their affiliated physicians. Beth Israel, on the other hand, purchased private, primary-care physicians' practices for the same reasons. Subsequently, Pathway was absorbed by CareGroup, now the overarching parent company.

When the Beth Israel Corporation, Pathway Health Network and Mount Auburn merged, seven hospitals were united and there were 10,000 employees and 1,800 medical staff, and it became one of the largest organized networks in the Northeast. Beth Israel Deaconess Medical Center would encompass both hospitals' campuses in the Boston Longwood Medical Area. Dr. Rabkin noted that this merger would allow them to offer increased high-quality patient care. Dr. J. Richard Gaitner said that the founding institutions' diversity and abilities gave the network strength.

The similarities between the two hospitals encouraged optimism about the merger. Both shared an affiliation with Harvard Medical School and the triple mission of patient care, medical education and research. Clinical expertise and respect for individuals were the underlying philosophies of each hospital and each retained its original religious roots. The early Beth

Israel had provided an institution wherein Jewish physicians and nurses could practice and Jewish immigrants would receive quality care with attention paid to their language limitations and dietary needs. The Deaconess hospital, deeply rooted in the Methodist religion, was presided over by a female deaconess. Each hospital's legacy included a cadre of talented, volunteer women who made major contributions to the hospital's growth and development and created a dedicated community of donors and trustees.

With the resignation of surgeons and anesthesiologists, BIDMC had difficulty recruiting new staff. Major, ongoing financial losses and staff dissatisfaction were widely publicized. Details of infighting, back stabbing and even negative clinical outcomes at BIDMC appeared in the media as insiders "dropped a dime" on their own colleagues. Other medical centers took advantage of the turmoil by aggressively recruiting Beth Israel Deaconess staff and patients. Some referring physicians began to shift their loyalties and patients to other hospitals. Angst continued at the senior staff level even after the initial departure of Deaconess chiefs. Battles were fought not only over how programs should be run but over who should run them. Restaffing and integrating two major departments (surgery and anesthesia) was truly an arduous task.

The drastic changes in the composition of the boards of trustees resulted in the loss of many venerable Beth Israel trustees whose status had been abruptly changed to that of non-voting "overseers." Now they were only welcomed at board meetings when invited. Most of the individuals had served on the Beth Israel board for decades and were the lifeblood and financial base of the hospital. They had experiential knowledge of the hospital and its history and identified strongly with Beth Israel, referring to it as "my hospital." With no notice, they received letters in the mail informing them of their removal from active board membership effective on receipt.

The dismissed trustees' anger and deep sadness might have been averted had they been forewarned and then notified of their change of status in a more personal and thoughtful manner. It was not what the board did but the manner in which it was done. Asked in 2003 about the cold, formal dismissal letter, Mr. Allan Rottenberg, president emeritus of the board, acknowledged its harshness but asserted that the change in status was necessary to form a more efficient board. He asked what the hospital could do now, several years after the fact. He then sidestepped the question, saying only that he favors compromise and tries to see all sides of an issue— and that it would be impossible for a fifty-member board to make timely, efficient decisions. He rejected the suggestion of a meeting at which the offended trustees would be offered a sincere apology by the current board with appreciation and gratitude expressed for their years of service and contributions. An apology goes a long way toward healing wounds. Mr. Rottenberg said such a meeting could not occur because of "legal complications."

The shake-up of the Beth Israel board took its toll on donations. The Combined Jewish Philanthropies had, in previous years, provided eighty percent of Beth Israel's operating revenue.

From 1994 to 2000, six presidents led the Beth Israel Deaconess. When Dr. Rabkin stepped down, Mr. David Dolins, a longtime member of Dr. Rabkin's senior management team, assumed the leadership but was unable to calm the waters. Dr.

Herbert Kressel, Dr. Michael Rosenblatt and Dr. Robert Meltzer followed, each remaining in office briefly. In 1999, after interviews with thirty-four candidates, Deaconess trustees urged the selection of Dr. James L. Reinersten. Mr. Kaye had previously known Dr. Reinersten, in earlier years, and when he appeared before the board they said that "He was it."

Despite the board's decision, from day one of his appointment, BIDMC administrators and physicians raised questions about Dr. Reinersten's suitability for the position. Prior interviewees and CEOs had brought their experience as Beth Israel staff or board members. Background knowledge had helped them seek strategies to improve the hospital's fiscal health without compromising its unique identity. Dr. Reinersten knew little of the two histories and disparate cultures that Beth Israel and Deaconess brought to BIDMC. In particular, he was unschooled in the philosophies that had shaped and guided Beth Israel including the value placed on close relationships among colleagues and the crucial role of primary nursing. One of the senior staff referred to Dr. Reinersten as "a brilliant visionary who was unfortunately difficult with people and could only relate to them from behind a lecturing podium."

Late in 1999, with Dr. Reinersten at the helm, CareGroup and BIDMC launched a new, strategic approach to turn around the hospital's financial performance. Plans included a fresh effort to compete with other Harvard hospitals, in particular the Brigham, for a larger share of the market and for the highest-paying medical procedures. BIDMC considered initiating a collaboration with a drug company, offering them first look at any new technological or pharmaceutical research. The third strategy was to raise millions of dollars by selling twenty percent of the medical center's real estate.

Selling hospital property would be a major, highly charged step for the trustees to take. However, the intent was that millions of dollars would be raised by selling twenty percent of the medical center's space. This not only included the sale of the Libby building, but they also contemplated selling the five-year-old, $1.2-million Shapiro Clinical Center. As the sales were initiated CareGroup considered eliminating some of BIDMC's clinical departments—psychiatry, dermatology and orthopedics—and moving those services to affiliated community hospitals. For example, New England Baptist, now a CareGroup hospital well known for orthopedic specialty services, would absorb orthopedic referrals from BIDMC. This plan would allow BIDMC to focus more resources on fewer high-level specialties.

The Boston Globe reported these planned changes, warning that they would seriously change the city's medical landscape. Though the *Globe* article provided no details about BIDMC staff reductions or clinical department closings, employees feared their jobs would disappear with the departments.

The buildings for sale not only had financial value but sentimental as well. Mr. Theodore Libby, a trustee, had helped Beth Israel buy a brick building on Brookline Avenue, joining a long list of Jewish philanthropists whose names are engraved on the hospital buildings. When asked by the *Globe* how he felt about the sale, he said, "The important thing is the survival, security, and well-being of the Beth Israel. What we were able to do at one point in time, donating the building, is fine but if it no longer serves a purpose, it should be sold. The hospital is a lot more important than

Shirley and Theodore Libby." His original donation stipulated that if the building were sold or demolished, there would be a suitable replacement "such as a plaque that would acknowledge our contribution to the hospital." Now two bronze plaques are affixed on either side of the entrance to the Shapiro building engraved with the names of Theodore Libby, his wife and his children.

Mr. Theodore Berenson, a former trustee and a real estate executive, had donated funds for the Berenson Emergency Services Unit in the 1970s. Asked how he felt about the sale, he said that he would continue to support the hospital—and that the changes being made were sound strategy. He remarked that his mother had lived across the street from Beth Israel's original building and his family had been involved long before he'd donated funds for the emergency room.

A BIDMC building at 21 Autumn Street was sold to Children's Hospital. The Kennedy building on the Deaconess campus was also sold. The Shapiro Clinical Center on Longwood Avenue, the newest of the hospital's buildings, was considered. Its loss alone would reduce BIDMC's space by twenty percent. The institute for training young physicians, medical offices and a multi-level, underground garage were irreplaceable. Parking in the Longwood area is virtually impossible. The garage was a most valuable asset to BIDMC, providing parking space for the community, the staff and the hospital's patients. Recognizing its value, the board rescinded its decision to sell the Shapiro building.

As part of the overall cost-cutting strategy, in 2001, the Care-Group board and Dr. Reinersten closed the 116-year-old Waltham Hospital, a distinctly unpopular move. Until its last days, Waltham served its local community, particularly with the provision of maternity services, which were heavily utilized. Its several-million-dollar losses convinced the CareGroup board to shut the hospital's doors. This was a significant loss to the local community. One trustee cited insufficient Medicare and Medicaid reimbursement as the primary reason for the closure. Others complained that CareGroup did not force the hospital to implement cost-cutting measures. Several years later, the CareGroup board voted to restrict their own authority over the clinical practices and the spending at affiliated hospitals.

The Waltham hospital's closing exhibited the CareGroup board's power and control. In order to close the hospital, the CareGroup board first had to disband the hospital's local board, whose closing they vehemently opposed. Five years later Mr. Levy discussed the Waltham Hospital closing in his online blog: "This use of reserve powers by the holding company board sent a shockwave throughout the system. While everyone knew the CareGroup board could exercise their authority, it had never been used so dramatically."

Given the continuing loss of millions of dollars by BIDMC, three very expensive consultants were hired. All highlighted the issues needing attention; each provided different plans. The Hunter Group, known in the community as "crash and burn consultants," proposed BIDMC staff be cut by 150 nurses and 268 physicians.

In 2000, two days before Christmas, Dr. Reinersten issued an order for an emergency, two-day retreat that would meet twelve hours each day. Mr. Levy, then administrative Dean of Harvard Medical School, attended the retreat, which included medical administrators and board members. Later, he recalled that at the retreat they were able to generate a good vision statement as well as plans for improvement and details of the work that needed to be done. At the time Mr. Levy was optimistic. Yet as time passed and he saw no evidence of the plan's implementation, he began asking what happened to the agreement. The responses from Dr. Reinersten were vague—they were revising the plan, or the administration didn't like it. Then, there would be silence. Mr. Levy felt that the CareGroup and BIDMC management did not welcome his input and he found this frustrating since nothing was being done. "This was not a question of not knowing what to do," he recalled. "Everyone knew what had to be done."

Dr. Reinersten's stated goal was to reduce the corporation's losses and debt while increasing its income. Yet he was the second-highest-paid hospital executive in Boston. His starting salary in 1999 was $803,400, including $83,437 for moving expenses. That same year, Beth Israel reported a loss of $130 million.

Besides his failure to move BIDMC into the black and throughout his tenure, Dr. Reinersten gave no evidence of understanding the hospital's internal problems wrought by the merger. Dissent and anger remained among staff with no leader to stem, address or relieve the tension. In fact Dr. Reinersten's demeanor kept people at a distance and was the prime contributor to the negative atmosphere, antagonism and conflict. Many members of the staff said that Dr. Reinersten's personality and leadership style were his undoing. One of his mottoes was, "Don't bring me your problems. Bring only solutions." Several interviewees referred to him as "an empty suit." Another said that when exiting his office, she felt as though she'd walked out of a refrigerator.

One staff member said that Dr. Reinersten looked good on paper but could not relate on a human level. The tolerance for missteps was very limited, said Dr. Kressel, a former Beth Israel CEO.

He could talk a good game but couldn't "walk the walk." Another vice president, Dr. Richard Wolfe, director of the emergency department, said, "Decisions happen and they happen quickly. That's the difference with the current regime."

At a meeting of senior staff discussing budget cuts in the obstetrical department, Dr. Henry Klapholtz, an obstetrician known for his even temper, said that Dr. Reinersten was destroying the hospital. The room, filled with physicians, applauded. Each staff member interviewed in 2003 and 2004 commented on Dr. Reinersten's lack of people skills. He was a misfit at Beth Israel. He had no tolerance for sentimentality. If one spoke of the "good old days of the BI" his response was, "It will never be the same. GET OVER IT." This was a time when staff were grieving, reminiscing, sharing memories and perhaps were also lamenting their own youth and the loss of colleagues.

A partner of the prestigious law firm Hale and Dorr said that there should be a total restructuring of the assets on Longwood Avenue. Dr. Reinersten disagreed, saying that putting all the Harvard hospitals together was impractical. He predicted that CareGroup would at least break even by fiscal 2002. Yet BIDMC lost $73 million in 2001. Financial losses, combined with declining patient volume, prompted Standard & Poor's to downgrade CareGroup's bond rating to minus B from triple B+.

To increase income and market share, Dr. Reinersten arranged for BIDMC to purchase private, primary-care medical practices with the expectation that referrals from these practices would increase BIDMC admissions. Not so. It was said that the hospital overpaid for the practices and at times had to subsidize them. Mr. Levy, who succeeded Dr. Reinersten as CEO, later reflected that the purchase of several private-practice physicians groups had not succeeded because the hospital had paid too much for the practices and created incentives between the community doctors and the hospitals that were improper .

Dr. Reinersten was fired July 2001.

From then on, with Mr. Robert Meltzer serving as CareGroup's interim CEO, the hospital began to right itself and finally allow BIDMC to realize some benefits of the merger. Mr. Meltzer was committed to measures that would enable CareGroup to compete against Partners. He had three tasks: to create a search committee for a new CEO, to break down the antipathy that continued to exist between the administrative and medical staffs and to create a steering committee to assist him in reducing the organization's financial problems.

To tackle the problem of surgeon recruitment, Dr. Josef Fischer, a nationally recognized surgeon, was hired as a consultant to assess the surgical department. He said, "You've got two full hospital surgical divisions. There is free-floating anxiety and morale problems. To make matters worse, while academic medical centers generally have a hard time recruiting surgeons, it is even more difficult in Massachusetts, where fees from managed care companies are low, balanced billing illegal, and the cost of living especially high."

Dr. Michael Zinner, chief of surgery at Brigham, said that even though the Harvard name was well respected, no one was going to come for the name alone. Dr. John Mayer, cardiothoracic surgeon at Children's Hospital, noted that not everyone considered Harvard the place to be—especially doctors who would have to take a thirty-percent pay cut and live in an area where the cost of living was fifty percent higher.

Part of Dr. Fischer's challenge was that while Harvard Medical School affiliation might have attracted some doctors or professors, remuneration was priority. In 2004, the salary included a cap of $532,000. To exceed the cap, hospital managers required permission from their own boards and the Dean of Harvard Medical School. Now, the BIDMC chief of surgery more than fulfilled expectations in his recruitment of highly qualified surgeons from throughout the country.

The adequacy of due diligence was an ongoing question. In March 2002 Dr. Rabkin spoke at the Massachusetts Institute of Technology Workplace Center's Conference on Enhancing Patient Care Through Enhancing Employee Voice: Reflections on the Scanlon Plan. Asked about due diligence in the question-and-answer period, Dr. Rabkin said, "In an ideal world, due diligence should not only deal with the finances of the two organizations that are merging but the way things are done and the history of the two. You say this is part of the package. This is the way we do it and this is the way we are going to do it because two organizations will use the same words with markedly different meanings."

Preparation had not been anticipated for dealing with underperforming subsidiaries. At the time of the merger, CareGroup owned the five community hospitals that belonged to the Deaconess parent corporation, Pathway, as well as the hospitals and providers that were owned by Beth Israel. Few were producing the desired income. The combined losses were the obligation of all CareGroup entities and had to be shared by all. In 1996, animosity was engendered when CareGroup required the profitable New England Baptist and Mount Auburn hospitals to subsidize corporate losses at a significant cost.

In 1996 Mr. David Dolins was promoted to replace Dr. Rabkin as CEO/president. When interviewed in 2003 he assumed blame for urging Dr. Rabkin, who was ambivalent about the merger, to go along with it. Initially, he and Dr. Rabkin had expected that Beth Israel would take over the Deaconess. Mr. Dolins said that the merger had been "the most horrible event he'd ever participated in." Now, more than ten years later, Mr. Dolins still feels guilty for having pressured Dr. Rabkin. Once the merger was accomplished, Mr. Dolins thought Dr. Rabkin did not take a sufficiently firm position with the newly reconfigured board of trustees—an entity that reflected greater Deaconess influence than did Beth Israel management and staff. The board was "totally uncooperative and unsupportive of the management team," Mr. Dolins said. Trustees from the Beth Israel board "seemed more interested in being buddy-buddy with the Deaconess trustees than maintaining the Beth Israel quality and image." Another senior executive said, "The board broke trust with the administration, staff, and employees. It will be hard to restore."

Dr. Rabkin and his team realized that the CareGroup board, now comprising Beth Israel and Deaconess trustees and recent appointees, rejected the consensus mode of resolving issues. Clearly, the extraordinary restructuring of both boards was ineffective in integrating toward a single purpose. With agendas hidden, there was no guarantee that the board and management would remain aligned.

Dean Tosteson was invested in and committed to a successful merger. With the agreement of the Harvard hospitals, he appointed Mr. Levy to the CareGroup steering committee in August 2001. This was the first time Dean Tosteson had placed a member of his own staff in a managerial role at a Harvard hospital. The CEOs of all the Harvard hospitals had no objections.

When interviewed in 2003 Mr. Levy said that had he been in charge of the merger, he would have focused on back-office issues rather than clinical functions, to take advantage of opportunities to achieve administrative gains and reduce duplication. He said that the merger was intended to solve management problems, not health care or medical issues. Instead of demotions or firings he would have waited for retirements or resignations.

His assessment was that the continuing financial failure of BIDMC resulted from a loss of volume. "They were overstaffed, short on vision, had a surplus of physical space, and poorly executed contracts with insurance companies. This was not a question of not knowing what to do but was a failure of leadership and governance. The board of directors did not have their fingers on the pulse of the organization and failed to set clear objectives or hold management accountable."

Some staff and trustees of the former Deaconess Hospital reminded one of burn victims when they talked about the merger. They felt that the Beth Israel had taken over the Deaconess and one can easily see how their experience might validate this perception.

A gentleman known as "the institutional memory of the Deaconess" has been a valued volunteer for more than fifteen years. When he heard of this project, he initiated a telephone conversation with the author but refused to be interviewed. Clearly, he was distressed and very angry, and referred to the merger as a "dirty takeover." Angrily, he asked, "Why would anyone want to go into that history? Why would they want to drag that up? People are just beginning to get over it." He didn't want the wounds reopened and doesn't want to dredge up unpleasant memories. "Forget the past. What are you going to do with a book? Hide it in the Weidner Library? Give it to patients? We'll lose patients. They don't want to go to a hospital that has troubles." He added that their "big mistake was not paying attention to the differences in culture. Many people were wounded and I'm not going to talk about the truth of the merger and make them reexperience all that pain. I don't look to the past. I look to the future."

Efforts to explain the book as an oral history provided him no comfort. Very few people associated with the Deaconess staff, administration, or trustees were willing to be interviewed. Their remaining feelings of pain and anger were instantly palpable when discussing the merger. Unfortunately this interfered with a more equally balanced story; forty-six people associated with Beth Israel willingly participated in interviews as did three members of the Deaconess.

Mr. Donald Lowry, president emeritus of the Deaconess for more than twenty years (1954-1975), was interviewed in his home. His history with the hospital and staff is replete with accolades not only because of his accomplishments but becuse of his long-standing, close relationships with all levels of staff. He discussed with pride the achievements of the Deaconess and its contribution to outstanding health care delivery for more than a century. He spoke of the loss of old friends and particularly grieved the loss of Dr. Gaitner, a friend of many years. Shortly after the merger, Mrs. Ames, a longtime friend, bequeathed an unrestricted gift of $18 million to the Deaconess. Mr. Lowry said, "The funds went directly to the Beth Israel" and he knows of "no benefit accruing to the Deaconess." He had hoped some of the money would have underwritten the naming of a building for her, or at least a part thereof. His parting words were, "This was a merger of last resort. The Beth Israel took over the Deaconess," and, "Dr. Rabkin is a man of integrity and a straight-talker."

Dr. Richard Gaintner died on May 28, 2004. Dr. Rabkin was quoted in *The Boston Globe:* "I don't think there was a hostile bone in his body. Everybody liked and thought well of him." Mrs. Gaintner said, "He had a real desire to make the health care business more humane."

An interviewee who requested anonymity was a former president of the Deaconess board. In 2003 he spoke of his resentment of Beth Israel because Dr. Gaintner was "such a kind man, beloved by all." He had to step down in favor of Dr. Rabkin. Though he considered Dr. Rabkin a "highly intelligent man who had a loyal staff and charisma," this gentleman felt as though Dr. Rabkin was not equipped to deal with the new, different, difficult problems confronting the hospitals and became arrogant and inflexible.

Had Mr. Levy led Beth Israel Deaconess from the start, the merger might have evolved quite differently. Dr. Rabkin, trained as a physician, was a creative thinker whose values and commitment to health care delivery were unsurpassed. He turned a small, ethnic hospital into a nationally recognized medical center. Mr. Levy, trained in urban studies and public policy, served as the effective manager of many complicated projects in the public sector, chairing the department of public utilities during an energy crisis, and then became head of the Massachusetts Water Resources Authority with a mandate to clean up Boston Harbor. That he did, and completed the project in advance of the deadline and below budget.

The merger having survived more than a decade, Beth Israel Deaconess has successfully survived Partners HealthCare and a near-death experience. Though Mr. Levy's decision making is not driven by consensus or sentiment, his management style is decisive, and he appears to be well considered and focused on the well-being of the hospital. Services have increased; combined, BIDMC is stronger and successful with the ledger, no longer in the red. Eminently clear, his thoughts and plans for the delivery of health care are at the pinnacle. His office door is literally always open. Obviously, he did not follow Dr. Donald Berwick's advice to "blow up" the health care system.

Both Mr. Levy and Dr. Rabkin are not only brilliant but also deeply invested in the Beth Israel Deaconess and patient care. Their styles of management differ, however: Dr. Rabkin is known for decision making by consensus while Mr. Levy is "hard-nosed" and avoids second-guessing himself. Instead, he makes and then implements a decision. If plan A fails, he goes to plan B. His decisions are for the good of the hospital. Sentimentality and people's feelings are not the determinants in his decisions. He, too, has a talent for hiring the best and the brightest. With a corporate mentality, he is self-confident and has every expectation that he will be successful in stabilizing the hospitals. He is said to be politically sophisticated, an impressive negotiator, and has the respect of all the leaders of the Boston medical institutions.

Chapter 9

A Man for All Seasons

"The great pleasure in life is doing what people say you can't."
—Walter Baghot

When Mr. Paul Levy was appointed president and CEO of BIDMC on January 7, 2002, he was taking on a health care system that had been redefined, reorganized and globalized into an industry that had been far beyond imagination ten years earlier. He enjoyed a solid reputation as the effective administrator of the Boston Harbor cleanup, a filthy body of water that had attracted national attention. In the 1960s a rock group, The Standalls, had released their ode to Boston Harbor, entitled, "Dirty Water." This same song was used as an effective tool that maligned then-governor Michael Dukakis when he ran for president in 1988. At that time Paul Levy, executive director of the Massachusetts Department of Public Utilities, had his new mandate: orchestrate the mammoth Boston Harbor cleanup. Under his leadership the $8-billion project was completed under budget and ahead of schedule.

In 2005 Joseph Favaloro, executive director of the Massachusetts Water Resources Authority Board, spoke of Mr. Levy's creativity, saying, "He seemed to pull solutions out of his hat." However he also believed that Mr. Levy "spent too freely and too fast on the project leading to double-digit water rate increases that outraged rate payers." He also said, "Paul was willing to get into the middle of the fray and fight it out." Among his various administrative skills he had the ability to make harsh decisions without apology, which proved to be an essential asset in managing the problems faced by the Beth Israel Deaconess Medical Center. In a 1998 *Boston Globe* interview, Mr. Levy said, "I like industries in transition or in turmoil. As much as I enjoy consulting, there's nothing like actually trying to get something done with your own team." When interviewed for this book in 2006, he said, "Problems are fun."

He prides himself on being a tough and effective negotiator, saying he "makes few promises and fulfills them." Blunt, outspoken, and self-confident, he said, "I can do almost anything I put my mind to." He was well aware that the challenges of health care delivery in the early twenty-first century were formidable, painful and complicated. These choices had to be made without sacrificing the conflicting needs of financial viability and patient care. In 2001 *The Boston Globe* reported on the fiscal status of the major Boston hospitals and noted that four of the six CareGroup networks had lost $76.7 million the previous year. At the same time Partners posted a $48-million operating gain.

For the first five years post-merger, the staff fought over issues large and small amidst toxic cultural clashes. Many millions of dollars were lost and the combined institutions were on the brink of insolvency. While the original intent of the merger was to strengthen the two hospitals, instead it nearly destroyed them. Mr. Levy announced, on his first day in office, that the days of indecision were over and sent a memo to each employee asserting that they had one last chance to save the Beth Israel Deaconess. That same week he hired the Hunter Consulting Group to analyze the hospital's problems and offer solutions. An assembled team of auditors rapidly generated a final report proposing massive cuts in staff: 625 people. On the chopping block were 150 nurses and 268 physicians. Though firing them would have reduced the massive flow of red ink and addressed the immediate budgetary issues, it might also have interfered with the level of care required to maintain services and the hospital's stellar reputation. By rejecting their recommendations, the nursing department remained at current levels.

Paul Levy said that problems, conflicts and challenges arose because of cultural differences and management styles. Beth Israel, renowned for its primary nursing, had a low patient-to-nurse ratio. Nurses were held in the highest esteem and had greater empowerment in decision making for their patients than Deaconess nurses who, though highly valued, took their orders directly from physicians. Though publicized as a merger of equals, it was in fact a takeover of the smaller, specialized Deaconess hospital by Beth Israel.

A 2002 study prepared by Price Waterhouse Coopers for American Health Insurance Plans examined the factors contributing to the rising national health care costs and analyzed where and how the health dollars were spent. They reported a ten-percent increase in medical liability costs, and health insurance premiums rose 8.8 percent between 2004 and 2005. Some physicians practiced defensive medicine, ordering expensive tests and prescribing high-priced medications perhaps more for their own protection against malpractice suits than primarily for the patient's benefit.

Referrals to specialists were sometimes made to avoid accusations of negligence. In 2002 the Bureau of Labor Statistics stated that one percent of the most seriously ill patients accounted for twenty-five percent of total health care expenditures. The top fifty prescriptions brought in revenues of just over $2 billion.

A bitter dose of medicine including layoffs, cutbacks and other painful measures accelerated the implementation of Mr. Levy's "turnaround plan." Anticipating that fierce battles might ensue, he established rules of engagement and solicited staff's help in devising solutions. Everyone was free to criticize his plan and he expected them to offer reasonable alternatives. While his assessment may have shocked some employees, he thought many were actually relieved now that the problems were openly discussed, not hidden. E-mails were sent to his office by the hundreds, many of which he personally answered. He said, "From that point forward everything is going to be out in the open. I have no choice. The whole city is watching. The issues of hospitals have nothing to do with medicine and health care. They are management, organizational and business problems."

The hospital administration had a static view of a dynamic process. They were moving targets and required constant vigilance to anticipate the next federal mandate and be prepared to make rapid, preemptive decisions. Like ships at sea, hospitals had to be ever-vigilant of the local climate and anticipate precipitous changes that could wreak havoc. He understood that the health care system rested on shifting sands with unforeseen barriers.

Despite the precarious financial situation in 2004, Beth Israel Deaconess made an unprecedented investment in the department of surgery by providing Dr. Josef Fischer, the newly appointed chief of surgery, the funds to recruit and hire surgeons. Replacing the forty surgeons lost in the aftermath of the merger reestablished the department of surgery. At about this time, Mr. Levy forged a $2.5-million marketing contract with the Boston Red Sox, becoming the team's official hospital.

How would the newly overhauled administration proactively anticipate new challenges, sustain the bottom line and increase bargaining power without restricting or compromising services? While providing quality services to the ever-increasing elderly and uninsured population there was concern that a clarion call for rationing might be triggered. The rising costs of medical insurance, reimbursement limitations to physicians, hospitals and the medical "arms race" confronted all but a few Boston hospital administrators. When Paul Levy was asked why he'd accepted such an arduous job, he said that it was a public service and that along with the Dean he was determined to save the hospital.

His task was daunting. Under intense public scrutiny he had to save the complex, a rapidly failing organization whose culture was marred by indecision and distrust. According to Paul Levy, when fundamental changes occur in hospital administrations, as they did in 2002 at BIDMC, the executive staff and board of trustees undergo dramatic changes in the constituency.

Many of the loyal senior administrative staff and decision-makers found themselves relegated to small, back-corridor offices. Mr. Levy said, "Loyalty may actually be an encumbrance to change. Regardless of seniority and loyalty, if a senior staff member is fired, you don't alert them in advance of their removal. When they arrive at work on Monday, their office lock has been changed." Retaining senior staff may in fact cause dissension, half the staff with the incumbent and the other half with the charismatic new leader.

When medical institutions experience a significant turnover of senior management, staff's resistance to change and uncertainty of leadership is by far one of the most difficult challenges to be confronted. Mr. Levy's history and determination in the face of previous trials and complex problems made it eminently clear that changes would occur but stability would prevail. His explicit plans and expectations were not only articulated but reinforced by his actions. When dealing with medical and operational problems, he blended a heavy dose of discipline with public reinforcement and he developed guidelines for behavior with the demand that everyone in the hospital measure up to them.

BIDMC decision makers had to adopt the most beneficial fiscal plan for the hospital. Mr. Levy's Turnaround Plan focused on accountability with a business plan similar to that of Harvard Business School models. Included were measurable targets, investment plans with projected returns on investments and the efficacy of a given program. Therefore administrations had to be prepared and ever-watchful for the next government mandates or restrictions. Developing new and effective strategies were required to avoid the ongoing proliferation of hostile and punitive actions by competitors against staff and the hospitals while providing quality services to the rapidly increasing elderly and underinsured population.

Massachusetts reaps significant benefits from high-quality medical care, particularly in Boston, Worcester and Springfield, where academic hospitals are the principal providers of inpatient and outpatient care. Out-of-state residents, university students and low-income and unemployed patients heavily utilize their facilities.

On November 19, 2003, just ten months after Mr. Levy assumed his position, he devised a comprehensive strategic plan that was distributed throughout the hospital. In the introduction, he wrote: "We face private and governmental insurers that do not reward institutions for the kind of medical advances that are essential to our core mission. The state government continues its disgraceful, chronic underpayment to all providers for a safety-net health coverage and even the federal government is fickle in its desire to properly finance Medicare coverage. Our task is to chart a path for BIDMC that recognizes the health care environment for what it is. We must believe that what we do is so special that we cannot abide the thought of this institution being gone or absorbed into another corporation."

He adds, "If we were to measure ourselves against the performance of the health care industry in Massachusetts, we could easily settle on breaking even as a measure of success. Approximately half the hospitals in the state fail to do that."

The strategic plan detailed all aspects of the finances, imperatives and goals. He boldly established minimum targets such as "increasing our net assets by $100 million by the close of fiscal year 2007." He said, "It takes ten years for a merger to work." Once again he accomplished his plan ahead of schedule.

Interrelated problems brought on by federal mandates, health maintenance organizations and pharmaceutical companies all significantly impacted and interfered with the health care system. Since 1986, the average payment for malpractice claims rose from

$32,000 to $95,000 in 2002. Insurance companies were the largest beneficiaries, with attorneys close behind.

Tort reform, a hot-button issue, is one of the most conflicted and contentious national issues in the forefront of public policy. The expanding movement attempts to reshape the system by which consumers can access the courts for their right to sue and restrict the malpractice awards they receive. In 2002 the underlying malpractice litigation system moved from a back-burner simmer to a front-burner boil. To curb the growth of rapidly rising premiums, congressional bills suggest reduction of the statute of limitations on claims, attorney fees and limits of liability for malpractice injuries.

National medical organizations have launched an effort to persuade state and federal lawmakers to intensively address medical malpractice tort reforms, which establish significant limits on the size of legal awards to injured patients, limitations of fees lawyers receive in contingency cases, statutes of limitations and liability for the manufacture of certain products. The medical lobby claims that an avalanche of medical malpractice lawsuits has led to the dramatic inflation of physicians' malpractice insurance premiums and bears responsibility for a significant portion of the double-digit inflation in health care costs.

The rising cost of premiums for malpractice insurance and limiting payments to physicians and hospitals both add to the struggle with the medical arms race that confronts most hospital administrations. According to *Black's Law Dictionary*, economic damages are defined as the "funds used to compensate the plaintiff for the monetary costs of injury such as medical bills or loss of income." Malpractice is defined as "failure of one rendering professional services to exercise that degree of learning commonly applied under all the circumstances in the community by the average, prudent, reputable member of the profession with the result of injury, loss, or damage to the recipient of those services or to those entitled to rely upon them." Statute of limitations specifies "the period of time after the occurrence of an injury or, in some cases or its cause during which any suit must be filed."

While tort reform has had some success in a few states, proponents are working at the federal level to enact specific laws dealing with class-action lawsuits and medical malpractice. In 2006 the Congressional Budget Office stated that tort reform would do little to decrease health care costs. They claimed that cyclical patterns in the insurance market and lower yields from investments played major roles in the recent rise of malpractice insurance premiums. The report also stated that very few medical injuries become the subject of tort reform since it primarily refers to catastrophic injury cases and only to certain types of damages. Opinions on reform are bitterly divided. The Internet, however, is rife with blogs primarily in opposition to tort reform.

A sweeping overhaul of the class-action suit process was passed by Congress and signed by President Bush in February 2007.

Efforts to enact a national health policy have been a staple of presidential politics for decades. In the 1930s Franklin Delano Roosevelt wanted to enact a universal health insurance plan, as had Theodore Roosevelt during his failed presidential bid in 1912. However he feared opposition from the American Medical Association and the state medical societies. Harry Truman had the same idea only to meet resistance from union leaders concerned that members' benefits would decrease under a national system. Twenty-five years later, President Nixon proposed an employer mandate to insure workers. In the early 1990s President Clinton's health care task force was an utter failure.

President Bush urged Congress to pass a more restrictive and comprehensive medical malpractice reform bill in 2006 that was approved by the House but defeated by the Senate. That bill would allow limited, non-economic punitive damage awards to $250,000, place limits on time allowed for injured patients to file lawsuits and establish a contingency fee schedule for lawyers. A provision would also provide liability protection for pharmaceutical firms. Congress, however, has yet to agree on a comprehensive prescription drug benefit for seniors, fearing the cost would bankrupt the Medicare trust fund.

Secrecy permeated the entire health care system for many decades. It was their unstated coin of the realm. In contrast, Mr. Levy's beliefs and management style was transparency—the polar opposite. He insisted that physicians open honest dialogues with patients, clearly enunciating the costs of medical care and the services available to them. He considered secrecy and the withholding of information unacceptable. When he instituted his turnaround plan he agreed to participate in videotaped interviews, every two to four weeks, with David Garvin and Michael Roberto, faculty at the Harvard Business School. He provided them access to his daily calendar and reports that were in preparation for a multimedia study.

He said, "I wanted to get the unvarnished story as it unfolded. Students get to see what a leader does to execute a turnaround plan on a day-to-day basis." According to Drs. Garvin and Roberto, "Classroom response has been overwhelmingly positive. It also evokes a lot of emotion. The class is in awe of Levy but often splits after he fires the CEO… Students are uncomfortable with such a display of power."

His next assault on secrecy was to create a blog called *Running a Hospital*. He was the first hospital president to open a dialogue with the entire community. On January 18, 2007 Mr. Levy's blog headline was, "Do I Get Paid Too Much?" He posted his 2006 salary of $1 million and what followed was a flood of e-mail messages. A *Boston Globe* survey then listed the salaries of senior, nonprofit-hospital executives in Massachusetts: James J. Mongan, MD, Partners, $2.1 million; Elaine Ulian, $1.4 million at Boston Medical Center; John O'Brien, $1.3 million, U. Mass Memorial Medical Center; Dr. David Barrett, $1.3 million, Lahey Clinic; Dr. Mark R. Tolosky, $1.2 million, Baystate Medical Center; Dr. James Mandell, $1 million, Children's Hospital; Dr. Gary Gottlieb, $1 million, Brigham and Women's Hospital; and Peter Slavin, $1 million, Massachusetts General Hospital. When the BIDMC board of trustees were asked what they thought of the blog, Mr. Levy replied, "They think we are in the business of being honest with the public and transparent in what we do."

Not only did Mr. Levy receive local responses to his salary announcement but on April 8, 2007 four single-spaced pages in the business section of the Sunday *New York Times* displayed columns of "Executive Pay to Chief Executive's 2006 Compensation." Included in the list was base salary, cash bonus, perks, stock awards, options, total value of equity holdings, change in pension, deferment plan, lump sum pension, deferred compensation balance and the changes from the prior year. Approximately 250 additional directors of corporations/presidents were listed by name along with the incomes they received. Whether his forthright announcement triggered the above or it was coincidence is not known.

Transparency is a highly complicated concept for hospitals to embrace or even tolerate. The time had come for physicians to engage in open and honest dialogues with their patients, clearly enunciating the cost of care and services available to them. Mr. Levy considers secrecy or the withholding of information abhorrent. He recognizes that it not only heightens the risk of interpersonal conflicts between the caregiver and their patient but may impinge on the trust established between them. Sharing information and knowledge actually strengthens that bond and trust.

A recent study in *The Journal of the American Medical Association* reports that negative medical outcomes combined with poor patient-physician communication are basic ingredients for litigation. Encouraging open, bilateral communication enables patients to have appropriate expectations of their medical visits and physicians. Belief in the validity of transparency when expressed in a truthful and sensitive manner is at the core of meaningful relationships between a doctor and his or her patient.

Of necessity, transparency requires a commitment to honesty, integrity, forthrightness and veracity. The Clinton health care task force was a glaring example of secrecy that led to the shattering of their plan. The alliance of the Massachusetts General and Brigham and Women's hospitals exemplified the epitome of secrecy.

Price invades all levels of health care. In the 1940s and 1950s physicians set their own fees and patients paid for their care with dollar bills. Now doctors' fees are negotiated with insurance companies who have no alternative but to accept the rates that are apportioned for each group of physicians. The press reports that sixty percent of the public has difficulty reconciling health information, and the elderly are at an even greater disadvantage since many don't understand the language of medicine and certainly do not know what medical care actually costs. Now, Aetna, Inc., a major, national health care insurer, is posting online the prices of medical procedures negotiated with Cincinnati-area doctors.

Hundreds of medical procedures and tests are noted. Many plans continue high deductibles with tax-favored savings accounts, which consumers can use to pay for medical care once they've met their deductibles. Of course they must first know the cost of care and recognize that they must bear some of the burden of cost. It is assumed that insured patients will be charged the same prices for their out-of-pocket costs that doctors or hospitals would charge the insurer. Aetna says that prices vary from doctor to doctor depending on and including the prestige, scarcity or surplus of doctors in a given specialty or whether the doctor belongs to a small practice or a large medical group. All those factors directly affect price negotiations. The fees typically are discounted from the list prices that doctors charge uninsured patients and are available only to Aetna and its plan members. "To create a more functional health care market, we need transparency," says Ron Williams, Aetna's president.

While this is a step forward much of the success of such a plan is dependent on the medical, financial sophistication and education of the patient. Obtaining even basic price data is crucial, employers say. As consumer-driven plans rise in popularity, health insurers will compete less on premiums and more on the financial information of services. Mr. Timothy Cahill, president of My Medical

Control, a hospital chain with multiple locations, may charge 150 different prices for the same procedure.

Mr. Scott Atlas wrote in *The Wall Street Journal*, "When prices are openly stated and widely known, competition will ensue and prices will go down." He also said, "The idea of informed consumers knowing prices and controlling their health care dollar is extremely powerful."

On September 29, 2006 Mr. Levy wrote in his blog, "Hospitals and doctors don't get to set their own prices. They are negotiated with insurance companies." Recently, two CEOs of insurance companies in Massachusetts, Charles Baker of Harvard Pilgrim Health Care and James Roosevelt of Health Plan, were quoted in the press as being in favor of posting the prices that hospitals and doctors charge. Did they really mean that? This would mean that Harvard Community Health Plan and Tufts would have to disclose to the world the rates they have negotiated with BIDMC, Mass General, Tufts-New England Medical Center and the like in addition to the rates they pay different groups of physicians. In the past, sharing and the publication of these rates were not permitted and were actually in violation of antitrust laws. "Let me make it clear. We would love to have those prices made public because we believe it would make clear the largest player in our market, Partners Health-Care System (owner of MGH, Brigham and Women's Hospital and several others) get higher rates because of market dominance. We would rather have rates based on the quality of patient outcomes where the providers that achieve better results would be paid more." Maybe that is what "Jim and Charlie are hoping for too," so that consumers can make more rational choices about where to get their care. "Maybe they believe the best way to achieve it is for the state to order them to post their prices."

Paul, a responder on Mr. Levy's blog, wrote, "For insured patients, the responsibility to provide transparency should lie with the insurer. Since many health insurance policies have a lifetime benefit cap, patients who have such policies should care about their health care costs especially for the more expensive events like surgery and hospital stays."

By April 2005 more than 600,000 Medicare recipients were in test programs that pay doctors and hospitals bonuses for achieving better results. If the pay for performance fails, "The alternatives are far worse than anything we have now," said Dr. Michael A. Hillman, who oversees quality issues at Marshfield Clinic in Wisconsin. Under the current system many doctors see more patients, perform more tests, and conduct more procedures without regard to quality or results. To qualify for the bonuses, the doctor must save Medicare money by keeping patients out of the hospital and eliminating unnecessary procedures.

Many medical professionals say that Massachusetts is not an ideal place to practice medicine. The cost of living is very high and the deteriorating medical environment led to a shortage of physicians, low reimbursements for service, forbidden balance billing and preauthorization for imaging tests and prescription drugs. Even so, medicine continues to attract talented physicians who, through no fault of their own, are burdened with external pressure, frivolous malpractice suits or misuse of the system. The government's caveat is to determine reimbursement to hospitals and physicians, undermine some gains and create an environment of dissatisfaction. Now, many decades later, what insights have we gained?

Though the system is riddled with inefficiencies, excessive administrative expenses, inflated prices, poor management and waste, there are positives in health care delivery. However, as health care costs continue to rise, we are left to wonder why other advanced countries manage to spend much less than we do while getting comparable results. Paul Krugman, in a *Boston Globe* editorial, asserts that our health care system "drives a poor bargain with the pharmaceutical industry." He also notes that a large part of our health care expenditures is in paperwork. In a 2003 study in *The New England Journal of Medicine*, estimated administrative costs took thirty-one cents out of every dollar spent on health care, compared to seventeen cents in Canada.

Many issues continue to plague our health care system. For example, the high cost of vaccines precludes some children from being vaccinated. The lucrative financial ties of medical professionals to drug companies is a hidden windfall.

In July 2007 a new health care reform law was enacted in Massachusetts requiring all residents to purchase private health insurance. If they cannot afford even the least costly insurance, they will not be penalized but will have to resort to emergency rooms, forego care or accept hospitals' free care. National surveys found that more than half the consumers without coverage either forego care, or hospitals suffer the consequences.

Priorities shift, and anticipatory thinking and strategizing is vital. However, implementing change is often undermined by the secrecy of the Goliath hospitals. When secrecy is the modus operandi, smaller medical institutions are caught like deer in headlights. The rapidly increasing numbers of the aging population, chronic diseases and new drug-resistant illnesses all strain the health care system. Unanticipated new diseases, such as AIDs or a flu epidemic, and the aging of the Baby Boomers, may strain the system to its limits.

Lacking prophetic capabilities, the system is left to those creative, invested experts such as the national Institute of Medicine. A book written under their auspices, *Crossing the Quality Chasm,* offers an agenda and makes suggestions for the improvement of the system. They suggest that care be evidence-based, patient-centered and systems-oriented. The majority of health care resources are primarily used for chronic disease. They list ten new rules "to guide the transition to a health care system that better meets patients' needs":

1. Care based on continuous, healing relationships
2. Customization based on patient needs and values
3. The patient as the source of control
4. Shared knowledge and free flow of information
5. Evidence-based decision making
6. Safety as a system priority
7. The need for transparency
8. Anticipation of needs
9. Continuous decrease of waste of resources and patients' time
10. Cooperation among clinicians

Improving health care delivery is a monumental task in process. Though the task is daunting, much has been achieved in the past decade. Our constituency is becoming increasingly sophisticated about to medical issues and is beginning to recognize that only with the collaboration of the major players—government, medical professionals and the citizenry—do we stand a chance of reforming the system. Improving communications, increasing transparency of key stakeholders, the general public and the industry will provide opportunities for improvement. Would we be better off upending the entire system or concentrating on creating conditions that free the states to innovate on their own?

Bibliography

"Be careful reading health books. You may die of a misprint."
—Mark Twain

Aaron, John, MD	*The Future of Academic Medical Centers*	2001
American Medical Association	*Grand Rounds on Medical Malpractice*	1990
Angell, Marcia, MD; Random House	*The Truth About Drug Companies: How They Deceive Us and What to Do About It*	2004
Annas, George J.; Southern University Press	*The Rights of Patients: The Basic ACLU Guide to Patient Rights*	1989
Arras, John and Steinbeck, Bonnie	*Ethical Issues in Modern Medicine*	1999
Barry, John M.	*The Great Influenza*	2004

Bartlett, Donald L. and   *Critical Condition:*   2004
Steele, James B.;   *How Health Care in America*
Doubleday   *Became Big Business—*
                            and Bad Medicine

Benner, Patricia;   *From Novice to Expert:*   2000
Pearson   *Excellence and Power in*
                            Clinical Nursing Practice

Beth Israel Association   *Three Year Financial*   March 1975
                            Forcast and other
                            Information

Bok, Derek, MD   Speech at University
                            of Pennsylvania

Bruaer, Carl   *New England Deaconess:*   1999
                            A Century of Caring

Bystrainyk, Roman   "Curbing Corruption   April 2006
                            in Medicine";
                            Health Sentinel

Campo, Raphael   *The Poetry of Healing*   1997

Castleman, Benjamin,   *Massachusetts General*   1983
Crockett, David C. and   *Hospital, 1955-1980*
Sutton, S.B., Eds.;
Lippincott Williams & Wilkins

Clifford, Joyce C., PhD;   *Restructuring: The Impact*   1998
Jossey-Bass   *of Hospital Organization*
                                 on Nursing Leadership

Charlton, Earle Perry,   *The Charlton Story*   2001
Winius, George and
Clement, Richard;
Peter Lang Publishing, Inc.

Cushing, Harvey, MD   *The Medical Career*   1929

Feingold, David S., MD and   "Beth Israel Hospital   1970
Hiatt, Howard H., MD, Eds.   Seminars in Medicine";
                                 Archives of Internal Medicine
                                 126(3):527.

Flexner, James Thomas, MD;   *Doctors on Horseback:*   1937
Viking Press   *Pioneers of American Medicine*

Flugel, J. C.;   *Psycho-Analytic Study*   1921
The International   *of the Family*
Psycho-Analytic Press

Gaylin, Willard   "Faulty Diagnosis: Oct. 1993
                                 Why Clinton's Health-Care
                                 Plan Won't Cure What Ails Us";
                                 Harper's Magazine

Gawande, Atul; Picador	*Complications:* *A Surgeon's Notes* *on an Imperfect Science*	2003
Gordon, Suzanne; Back Bay Books	*Life Support:* *Three Nurses* *on the Front Lines*	1998
Herrick Smith Productions	"Dr. Solomon's Dilemma"; PBS *Frontline*	2000
Herzlinger, Regina; Basic Books	*Market Driven Healthcare*	1999
Institute of Medicine of the National Academies	*Crossing the* *Quality Chasm*	2005
	To Err is Human: *Building a Safer* *Health System*	1999
Johnson, Carolyn	"Influenza"; *The Boston Globe*	2004
Johnson, Haynes and Broder, David; Back Bay Books	*The System: The American* *Way of Politics at the* *Breaking Point*	1997

Kasden, Jack, MD	Interview with author	
Kastor, John A.; University of Michigan Press	*Mergers of Teaching Hospitals in Boston, New York, and Northern California*	2003
Kleinman, Arthur, MD; Basic Books	*The Illness Narratives: Suffering, Healing, and the Human Condition*	1989
Knowles, John H., Ed.; Harvard University Press	*Views of Medical Education and Medical Care*	1968
	Hospitals, Doctors, and the Public Interest	1965
Kowalczyk, Liz	"Brigham Struggles to Lure a Star Surgeon"; *The Boston Globe*	
Lange, Roger, MD	Interview with author	
Levy, Paul	*Running a Hospital*; runningahospital.blogspot.com	
Lieberman, Trudy	*Columbia Journalism Review*	Sept./Oct. 1993

Linenthal, Arthur, MD;
Beth Israel hospital
in association with
Countway Library
of Medicine, Boston, MA

First A Dream:
The History of Boston's
Jewish Hospitals 1896-1928

1990

Ludmerer, Kenneth M., MD;
Oxford University Press

Time to Heal:
American Medical Education
from the Turn of the Century
to the Era of Managed Care

1999

McCord, David;
Harvard University Press

The Fabrick of Man:
Fifty Years of the
Peter Bent Brigham Hospital

1963

McDermott, William V., MD;
Science History
Publications/USA

Surgery at New England
Deaconess Hospital

1995

McGrath, Patrick;
Knopf

Trauma

2008

Munson, Ronald;
Wadsworth Publishing
Company

Intervention and Reflection:
Basic Issues in
Medical Ethics

1979

Pekkanen, John;
Dell

M.D.: Doctors Talk
About Themselves

1990

Pendleton, James, MD	*Journal of American Physicians and Surgeons*	
Perkins, Lori	*Insider's Guide to Getting an Agent*	1999
Phillips, Susan S. and Benner, Patricia; Eds; Georgetown University Press	*The Crisis of Care: Affirming and Restoring Caring Practices in the Helping Professions*	1994
Porter, Michael E. and Olmsted Teisberg, Elizabeth; Harvard Business School Press	*Redefining Health Care*	2006
Rabiner, Susan and Fortunato, Alfred; W.W. Norton & Co.	*Thinking Like Your Editor*	2003
Rabkin, Mitchell, MD	Speech in East Room at the White House	June 27, 1994
Reuters	"Judge Lambeth Hearing"	March 1993
Rosenberg, Charles E.; Basic Books	*The Care of Strangers: The Rise of America's Hospital System*	1987

Ryan, Ethel Mascioli; Beth Israel Hospital Nurses' Alumnae Association	*Recaptured Memories: A Living History of Beth Israel Hospital School of Nursing, Boston, Massachusetts*	2001
Saal, Kim, MD	Interview with author	
Sandburg, Carl	"Washington Monument by Night"	
Sexton, Anne; Houghton Mifflin	*The Complete Anne Sexton*	1999
Sheehy, Gail; Random House	*Hillary's Choice*	1999
Starr, Paul, MD	*The Social Transformation of American Medicine;* Basic Books	1982
	The American Prospect	1994
	"The Signing of the Kennedy-Kassebaum Bill"; epn.org/library/signing.htm	Aug. 22, 1996
Tosteson, Daniel	Interview with author	
Various authors	*Newsweek*	

Bibliography

Various authors	*The Boston Globe*	
Various authors	*The Chicago Tribune*	
Various authors	*The Jewish Advocate*	
Various authors	*The New York Times*	
Various authors	*The Wall Street Journal*	
Various authors	*The Washington Post*	
Vogel, Morris J.; University of Chicago Press	*The Invention of the Modern Hospital, Boston, 1870-1930*	1980
Weinberg, Dana Beth; Cornell University Press	*Code Green: Money-Driven Hospitals and the Dismantling of Nursing*	2004
Williams, Stephen and Torrens, Paul R.; Cengage Learning	*Introduction to Health Services*	2001